Unheralded, lonely, and very hard—that's a *good* definition for caring for a loved one who struggles with disability. Every caregiver wonders, *Can I do this for the rest of my life?* Then, *Was this a big mistake?* And finally, *I'm trapped.* Despite all the good times in our thirty-eight years of marriage, I have felt the same. And it's why my wife Joni and I heartily endorse the book you hold in your hands. It's filled with bruising candor, honest stories, and heartwarming insights that will inspire and refresh the faith of *any* caregiver. Best of all, once you read this book, you'll realize, *I'm not alone!* So get reading, and be ready to be blessed!

KEN and **JONI EARECKSON TADA**, Joni and Friends
International Disability Center

This is a beautiful book. Jill Case Brown invites us into her story, her heart, and her soul. No simple answers, no easy formulas; Jill takes us on a journey of questions, weariness, anger, regrets, and renewal. As a former caregiver, I am hesitant to read books on caregiving by someone who has no "up close and personal" experience. I was drawn into Jill's story because of her honesty and raw emotion—because she's been there and is there

T0016839

all readers, to join her as she explores the hidden blessings God offers if one is open to journeying through the dark places of illness and caregiving. It has been a few years since my husband battled with, and died from, Alzheimer's disease, but *We're Stronger than We Look* blessed me with insight, wisdom, and words to assign to my still-present questions. This is a book for all current caregivers and for those who will become caregivers. I will keep several copies on my bookshelf, ready to gift to those in the caregiving community.

DR. CYNTHIA FANTASIA, author of *In the Lingering Light: Courage and Hope for the Alzheimer's Caregiver*

WE'RE
STRONGER
THAN WE
LOOK

Insights *and* Encouragement *for*
the Caregiver's Journey

JILL CASE BROWN

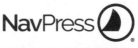

A NavPress resource published in alliance
with Tyndale House Publishers

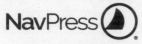

NavPress is the publishing ministry of The Navigators, an international Christian organization and leader in personal spiritual development. NavPress is committed to helping people grow spiritually and enjoy lives of meaning and hope through personal and group resources that are biblically rooted, culturally relevant, and highly practical.

For more information, visit NavPress.com.

For information about special discounts for bulk purchases, please contact Tyndale House Publishers at csresponse@tyndale.com, or call 1-855-277-9400.

ISBN 978-1-64158-388-6

Printed in the United States of America

28	27	26	25	24	23	22
7	6	5	4	3	2	1

For David's parents, Bob and Joan Brown, who said,

"We'll stay as long as you need us," and did.

CONTENTS

WELCOME TO YOUR BOOK

Does the walker choose the path, or the path the walker?

GARTH NIX, *Sabriel*

IF YOU HAVE BEEN, WILL BE, or are now a caregiver, this book is yours.

Or maybe you're checking to see if it might make a good gift for a caregiver you know. If so, that's great. Every caregiver needs someone like you in their life.

This is the book I would love to have been given when my husband, David, came home from the hospital as a new quadriplegic. Thanks to family and friends, we had good support. But then the time came for David's parents to head back to Delaware and for us to settle into life. I'd never liked the phrase "the new normal"—way too overused—but it kept popping into my mind. It fit our situation.

And here's the problem with that.

As a caregiver, your "normal" probably isn't like that

of most people you know. They can't really understand your world because they don't live in it. I didn't understand mine until I had to. Until then, I had no idea how many sidewalks bristle with broken concrete from tree roots or take scary, lumpy dives into and out of their intersecting alleys. I'd traveled those sidewalks how many times? Now, with David in a wheelchair, I see them differently: as challenges, obstacles, and sometimes impossibilities.

I love meeting people who do understand. It's good to talk, to compare experiences. But just when we most need that, we caregivers can't have it. We're at home, feeling isolated, overwhelmed, discouraged.

That's when we need a book written by someone from our world, and that's what this book is. I hope you find it both down-in-the-dirt real and a lift to your soul. It isn't a how-to. Instead, you'll enter into my life and the lives of other caregivers.

Depending on your situation, you'll probably connect with some chapters more than others. I hope you love them all. They're short because I know from experience that many caregivers have only brief spurts of time to read. But they should take you deep.

Be sure to read the quotes that begin every chapter.

Some might not have much meaning for you. But others suit their story so perfectly, they'll make you laugh, smile, cry, or whatever you need right then.

1

SHE'S GOT IT ALL TOGETHER

Comparisons are odious.

ANONYMOUS

SHEILA GLOWED WITH YOUTH AND LIFE. So did her husband, though his bulky power wheelchair somewhat cramped Tim's style. The four of us had arranged to meet for dinner at a restaurant, where we could trade stories and get to know each other.

Their how-we-met-and-married saga turned out to be as charming as they were. They'd known each other since kindergarten, but their casual friendship didn't deepen until after his diving accident. Tim waited a full year, wanting to make sure Sheila understood what she was getting herself into. Only then did he ask her to marry him, and she said yes.

"*I'll* say she did." Tim grinned. "She didn't even wait for me to finish the question."

Sheila grinned back. "I'd already waited too long."

Now, that's romance!

We in turn told about a cold January weekend when David and I led a marriage seminar at a downtown hotel. Back then, David could handle the three steps at our back door, so we didn't yet have a house ramp or converted van. To save time with our early morning start from home, I'd packed his manual wheelchair in the car trunk the night before. We got to the hotel, I assembled the wheelchair, and David sat down.

Thunk!

Overnight, his chair's gel cushion had frozen solid. To make matters worse, the heat malfunctioned in our part of the hotel. Everyone at the seminar was shivering—even those of us who didn't have to sit on a block of ice. The cushion took hours to thaw, and David never really warmed up that day.

Not romantic like their tale, but funny. Sheila laughed long and loud, then sighed and said, "I love stories like that."

After dinner, the four of us left the restaurant together. Tim and Sheila watched with interest as I helped David stand for his transfer into our car. The people from the SUV next to us showed up just then and stood around waiting for us to get out of their way. Flustered, I tried to hurry the transfer.

Sheila spoke up, her voice firm and confident. "Take your time. They'll wait."

Finally, David sat safely down on the passenger seat. I swung his legs in, closed the door, and hustled his wheelchair back to the trunk.

"G'night," Tim said. "Let's do this again. It's good to talk to someone who can relate."

"Definitely! This was great." Sheila hopped up to stand on the back of Tim's chair, holding onto its handles. She turned to wave at us and rode jauntily off to their van.

In the gathering darkness of the spring evening, their beauty pierced my soul. Tim and Sheila understood their challenges and met them with grace, youth, and clear thinking.

The SUV beside us drove away. Feeling dull, middle-aged, and foolish, I climbed into our trusty Chevrolet, buckled us both in, and headed for home. David and Tim might stay in touch, but I doubted Sheila and I would.

She had it all together. She didn't need me.

2

THE ELEPHANT
IN THE ROOM

Being able to laugh openly with friends is one thing;
feeling secure enough to cry openly with friends is quite another.

ERIC SANDRAS, *When the Sky Is Falling*

DAVID AND TIM DID STAY IN TOUCH. They talked by
phone every month or so, but the four of us didn't get
together again for another year.

That evening, we met at the same restaurant as before,
but the atmosphere around our table felt different. Tim
went on at length about his legal studies and a new
physical therapy he was trying. Sheila seemed quieter
than before, less ready to laugh. This was probably true
of David and me as well. All I remember is listening,
watching, and feeling vaguely uneasy. I don't recall how
the evening ended.

The next time David called Tim, we learned that Sheila had left him.

A year earlier, the beauty of their hope-filled story had pierced my heart. Now their affliction did the same. Sheila had believed she knew what she was getting herself into. But caregiving is hard.

Your friends plan a hiking trip. *That'll be fun. Sure wish I could go.*

Waking up tired, you face an hour-plus of hard work getting your person ready for the day. *Can I do this for the rest of my life?*

Then, *Was this a big mistake?*

And finally, *I'm trapped.*

Doubt. Resentment. Guilt. Shame. Fear.

It helps to have people around who understand. Why didn't Sheila call me? Maybe she had others to talk with. Or maybe she didn't know that's what she needed.

Why didn't I call her? What if I *had* called her? Would that have made any difference?

I don't have answers, but one thing I do know: Never again will I look at a caregiver and think, *They have it all together*. Because none of us do.

I dithered about this chapter. I almost didn't put it in. But my friend Jani, who cared for her mother for many years, said, "This is the elephant in the room for every caregiver. *What if I can't do this? What if I fail?* You have to get it out in the open."

She's right. So keep reading.

You may have come to caregiving as a profession, or circumstances may have thrust you into this work. In this book, when I refer to "your person," I'm referring to the human being on the other side of your caregiver relationship.

3

CONNECTING

Only two things pierce the human heart: beauty and affliction.
SIMONE WEIL

EVEN BEFORE MY HUSBAND broke his neck, I loved this quote by Simone Weil: "Only two things pierce the human heart: beauty and affliction." But after his accident, the words took on more meaning.

Beauty and affliction. As caregivers, you and I live in the center of both.

Sometimes we feel them pressing in at the same time, piercing us from opposite directions. Sometimes *we're* the beauty, though we may not feel like it. And sometimes we're part of the affliction.

Like the other night, when I was so tired I could almost taste sleep. All I wanted in life was to fall into bed and drag the covers up to my chin. First, though, I had to get David there. From clothes to pajamas, from wheelchair to bed. Then I had to change his external catheter.

He'd had a long day too. In the middle of the catheter change, he fell asleep and dreamed it was time to urinate.

Some dreams come true. This one did.

Thank you, God, for a washer and dryer in the basement. Thank you for extra sheets and pajamas, and for plenty of towels and washcloths. Thank you for your grace in the part I'd rather leave out. The part where I leaped around our bedroom, shouting out my disbelief and fury to my sleepy, startled, quadriplegic husband. I wish I *could* leave that out. I wish I hadn't done it. But I did.

I was so tired, God . . .

As for you, the caregiver reading this right now, I wish you could tell me your stories like this. Maybe someday you can; I hope so. In the twelve years since David took a violent header off his bicycle and into a wheelchair, I've learned that most caregivers love to hear each other's stories. We need them. We need to learn from each other. But more than that, we need the connection.

Think of how strings are knotted together to make a net. That's what caregivers are—a safety net, both as individuals and collectively. Because of us, people who can't care for themselves are lifted and held in safety all around the world. That analogy came to my mind the other day, and I think it suits.

Like a net, we belong to a loosely woven fellowship whose strands connect only at wide intervals. Ours is an enormous community, but its members hardly ever see each other. We can feel isolated, unsure, scared. It's often easy to see the affliction in how we live, while finding it hard to recognize the beauty.

But like a net, we're stronger than we look.

As of 2020, more than 1 in 5 Americans are family caregivers. That's an increase of 9.5 million since the last study (in 2015).[1]

4

THE DIVIDING LINE

Watch out for that first step; it's a doozy.

NED RYERSON, *Groundhog Day*

FLIPPING THE GARAGE KEY OFF its hook by the back door, I went outside. I undid the padlock and swung the old wooden door wide, ready for David to roll in on his bicycle. Then I walked down our gravel drive and looked both ways along the street, shading my eyes against the late-afternoon sun.

No David in sight.

Worried? No, not really. Let's call it a flick of uneasiness. He had a great commute on the path through the Garden of the Gods park, followed by a few blocks on a street with a clearly marked bicycle lane. Good and safe. I told myself he probably got caught up in a conversation as he left work. That could easily happen with our highly relational member care team. But it *was* getting late.

With a last glance at the street, I went back inside.

Rice and beans simmered on the stove. A handful of uncooked rice that had spilled from the bag crunched under my sandals. I fetched the vacuum cleaner and ran it over the kitchen floor. When I turned off the vacuum, the phone was ringing.

I snatched it up. "Hello—Browns."

The caller introduced himself. I remember that, though I don't remember his name. And he must have said he was a firefighter because I almost told him we had just given to their organization. But instead of a fundraising spiel, he said, "Do you have reason to be the emergency contact for a white male, late forties or early fifties, bicycling through Garden of the Gods?"

That's the part I remember most clearly. It marks the dividing line.

Half of me hung back from stepping over that line, still focused on the image of David coming home for dinner. The other half gripped the phone with both hands and said, "Yes, my husband. What happened?" Torn in two and suspended in time, I had to force urgency into the words. My voice sounded hollow to me. Unreal.

As the caller spoke again, the two halves swirled together. His words came in waves: "bike path . . . unconscious . . . no wallet, but we found his phone . . . can't get him to wake up."

The dividing line. When I hung up a few minutes later, I'd been dropped—or lifted—into a different life. Though I didn't know it yet, the hands that set the phone down, slowly and carefully, as if to make sure it didn't break, were now the hands of a caregiver.

God's hands. Beauty and affliction. Another strand in the safety net.

5

NOT WHAT YOU MIGHT EXPECT

Sundar Singh said, "What is science?"
"Natural selection and the survival of the fittest," he was told.
"Ah," Sundar Singh replied,
"but I am more interested in divine selection
and the survival of the unfit."

SUNDAR SINGH, *Reality and Religion*
(PARAPHRASED)

IN THE EARLY 1900S, Sundar Singh must have walked thousands of miles as a Christian missionary in the mountains of south Asia. Late one afternoon, he and a Tibetan guide pushed their way against icy winds on a high mountain pass. Darkness was coming on quickly. The guide warned Sundar they would certainly freeze to death if they didn't reach the next village before night.

As they struggled along, they came across a man who

had slipped from the narrow path and fallen downhill into deep snow. He was alive, but barely.

The guide refused to help Sundar rescue the man. "If we try to carry him, none of us will ever reach the village. We'll all freeze. Our only hope is to go on as quickly as possible, and that's what I intend to do. You'll come with me if you value your life."

Without looking back, the guide headed up the path.

Sundar couldn't bring himself to abandon someone who was still alive. He made his way down to the man, lifted him onto his back, and wrapped his blanket around them both. Climbing up again took a long time. As Sundar headed toward the village, swirling snow hid the steep path. Numb with fatigue but warm from exertion and their combined body heat, Sundar trudged through the falling darkness. Finally, he glimpsed houses a few hundred yards ahead.

Then he saw something on the ground beside him, nearly covered with snow. A person?

Slowly, keeping the man's weight balanced on his back, he knelt and brushed at the snow. Beneath it lay the body of the guide, who had frozen to death.

Years later, someone asked Sundar Singh, "What is life's most difficult task?"

He spoke without hesitation. "To have no burden to carry."

6

GOD'S HANDS

Nothing that is worth doing can be achieved in our lifetime.

REINHOLD NIEBUHR, *The Irony of American History*

As FAR AS I KNOW, Sundar Singh and our friend Mrs. Hastings never crossed paths. Too bad. I think they would have liked each other.

I met Mrs. Hastings during a visit to David's family, about a year after we married. She ran a small gift shop from her home, and David's mother had bought pewter bowls and plates for us there. Now Mother wanted to see if the shop had anything else we might like.

A double blessing. Nice things for the newlyweds, and income for old friends.

Mother had known Mr. and Mrs. Hastings since her teenage years, when he was her church's youth pastor.

He'd developed Parkinson's disease since then. His system couldn't tolerate the medications, and the disease overtook him. By the time I met them, Mr. Hastings was completely bedbound, and his wife had been his caregiver for more than twenty years.

"I'm so thankful I can have him here with me," she said as we stood in the little shop. "Come back to his room and say hello. He can't talk, but I know he'll be happy to see you."

I barely remember what he looked like. But each time I fill the pewter soup tureen Mother bought for us that day, I see Mrs. Hastings clearly, a tiny woman with short, gray hair and joyful eyes. *So* tiny. How could she possibly take care of a man who couldn't move on his own? After his death, Mother told me that in all the years his wife cared for him, he never had even a minor bedsore. That's amazing.

I spent only a few minutes with Mrs. Hastings that day, and not much more on later visits. But twenty-five years later, as I waited in the emergency room, it was her face, her name—and the things I'd heard Mother say about her—that came to mind. What she did carried beyond her lifetime and became a legacy for mine.

If Mrs. Hastings could do it . . .

Caregivers are God's hands, and not just to the person we're caring for. We give hope to people we don't even know are watching us.

7

AND SO IT BEGINS

Life is its own journey.

SIR LAURENS VAN DER POST, *Venture to the Interior*

THERE'S A GOOD CHANCE YOUR story started the same way mine did: The phone call. The white-knuckle drive to the hospital. And after that, hours and hours of waiting.

In the emergency room, my daughter and I waited with friends I'd called before leaving home. At first, we sat in the main area. Then they moved us to a small, private waiting room. I liked the privacy but not its implications. If you've been there, you know. Those rooms are meant for people likely to get bad news.

Our news came in trickles. David was still unconscious. The top of his helmet had cracked in half, but

X-rays showed no sign of brain injury. They did show a broken neck. He might live. He might not.

Restlessness jerked at my arms and legs. *Do something.* But there was nothing I could do.

Our daughter went outdoors to pace and cry and talk to friends on her phone. Then she came in and sat beside me, writing out everything she saw and heard and felt. When ER staff asked if we needed anything, she said, "Paper!" Puzzled but willing, they brought her some.

She kept writing. I kept twitching. I prayed, but everything in me seemed disjointed. I have no memory of the emotions I felt during those hours.

As the word spread, people called. Our friend Helen sat across from me, fielding calls on her phone and mine. The chaplain gave up on me and instead talked with Helen's husband, Ian, which was a relief. I just couldn't focus.

The doctor came again to tell us David's blood pressure was way too low and still falling. "We're losing him," he said. He stood to go, then asked, "Do you pray? Would you pray with me?"

Losing him. Losing him. Losing him. The words rolled like silent thunder beneath our prayers. As he left, he said, "If you have family, you should tell them to come."

I phoned David's parents again. I had just begun a stumbling explanation when the doctor sent word. While we were praying together, David's blood pressure had risen. He'd stabilized.

"Thank God," Dad said into the phone.

Stabilized. The first hint of a future, though probably different from what we'd known. With a faint but unmistakable sense of lifting, I thought, *If Mrs. Hastings could do it . . .*

I have no idea how much time passed before I finally got to see David. They warned me he still hadn't awakened, that he didn't look good. Bracing myself, I went in. The room looked as if a medical bomb had gone off, evidence of how fiercely the trauma team had fought to save his life. I picked my way through the debris and stood beside the gurney.

David. Face bloody and swollen, but definitely David.

Only then did I acknowledge that a small, stubborn part deep inside me had been waging its own fierce fight. Lobbying for this to be a mistake. Hoping to see a stranger lying on that gurney.

No mistake. No stranger.

Giving up false hope, I took a step into the real.

If Mrs. Hastings could do it . . . so can I.

8

WHEN HEROES GET PERSONAL

I think that we all do heroic things,
but hero is not a noun—it's a verb.
ROBERT DOWNEY JR.

EVER SINCE DAVID TAUGHT ME to look for quiet heroes, I've become more and more aware that we're surrounded by them. But their heroism *is* quiet. It rarely stands out. If publicity comes their way, they avoid it.

On the day of David's accident, heroes abounded. Just think of all those people at the hospital who daily hurl themselves into fighting for someone's life. That's what they do, and they're my heroes. They'll always be my heroes.

But that day, they weren't the first ones.

David had finished work that afternoon, hopped onto his bicycle, and headed home. He avoided the busyness of Thirtieth Street, instead staying on the trail that led down into Garden of the Gods park. A beautiful, peaceful commute.

Meanwhile, another cyclist was speeding along Thirtieth, above and parallel to David's route. Where the shoulder gave access to the trail, the cyclist swung sharply downhill. At a blind intersection formed by the slope, his path converged with David's.

No one knows exactly what happened there. But for a brief time after he finally woke up in the hospital, David remembered swerving to avoid a bicycle collision. Our boss walked the trail the next day to look for clues. He found David's badge lying near tire tracks that sheared off into sandy gravel. Any cyclist knows what that kind of surface can do to you. David had hurtled into the air and landed headfirst on a rock, crushing the first two vertebrae in his neck.

The other cyclist? We don't know. He probably kept going, unaware of what had happened just behind him.

A woman hiking the trail found David sprawled face down against the rock, not breathing. She scrambled up the hill and tried to flag down cars coming along Thirtieth. One pulled over, and she gasped out her story to the driver. "I think it's too late," she told him. "But please come."

The driver, a middle-school principal named John, had once done a short stint of EMT training. He followed her down the hill, calling 911 as he ran.

At first, he thought she was right: *Too late*. But then he found a faint pulse. He and a jogger who came along the trail carefully turned David faceup, supporting his neck. The jogger took over the phone, relaying the dispatcher's instructions as John did chest compressions.

When the EMTs arrived, David was doing agonal breathing: the gasping, last-ditch effort of a body whose heart had stopped pumping to somehow get oxygen to his vital organs.

No one thought he would live. Only God knows why he did.

To the woman who ran:

I know you were terrified when you
found David, convinced you stood

in the presence of death. You might have run away, pretending you hadn't seen. Instead, you ran for help and found the person God brought for that purpose. You did the right thing.

You didn't give your name, said you didn't want to know the outcome. But I wish I knew who you were. I wish you could know what you did for us.

Yours were the first hands. You were David's first caregiver.

The first of that day's quiet heroes.

9

TOTALLY UNQUALIFIED

Doing what is right is rarely the same as doing what is safe.

EDITH EVA EGER, _The Choice_

"_HERO_: A LARGE SANDWICH CONSISTING of a roll that is split lengthwise and contains a variety of fillings, [such] as lettuce, tomatoes, onions, meats, and cheese."[1] That scrumptious definition came out of my _American Heritage Dictionary_. It's accurate, but it doesn't exactly fit the heroes you met in the last chapter.

Neither do other suggestions under that listing. "Someone of great courage and strength . . . [who] does bold exploits . . . risks or sacrifices their life." No.

Or maybe yes.

Quiet heroes do have elements of those. The three people who kept David alive until the EMTs got there showed courage and strength. Their exploits *were* bold, in a quiet way. They risked possible failure, maybe a lawsuit if they messed up. They sacrificed time and effort, setting aside their own priorities in order to save David's life.

It would have been much easier to turn away. To say, "I can't. I'm not qualified to do this."

And that was true. They weren't qualified. I'm sure the reality of that thought loomed in their minds, which makes their actions even more heroic. The woman on the trail, her legs weak with fear, ran to get help. John, aware that his EMT training had been both brief and long ago, got out of his car and followed her. The jogger, sweaty and breathing hard, wiped his hands and reached out to help.

They stopped. They stayed. They did what was needed, when it would have been easier not to.

Maybe *that*'s my definition of a quiet hero.

I like it. Now let's add this to the mix: My definition of a quiet hero also describes *you*.

Think back to just before you became a caregiver. As you drove along your metaphorical version of Thirtieth Street, you probably had the next stretch of life planned out for yourself. A graduate degree, maybe. Moving up in your career. A chance to catch your breath, with the children all in school now. Fill in the blank; the possibilities are endless.

Then, need came pounding up the hill and flagged you down. And you stopped.

Did you have the qualifications to do what came next? I didn't. I don't know any caregivers who did, though there must be some. In many ways, it would have made sense for most of us to say, "I can't do this." Instead, we forced our scared, shaky legs to move us forward. We climbed out of our metaphorical car. We wiped our hands and reached out to help.

God's hands. Beauty and affliction. Another strand in the safety net. Quiet hero.

That's a caregiver. That's you and me.

I wish we could give each other a hug and a hero sandwich.

10

WOOF WOOF

---

saint (n.): a dead sinner revised and edited

AMBROSE BIERCE, *The Devil's Dictionary*

PART OF ME ENJOYS HAVING someone tell me what a selfless, loving caregiver I am, a saint with wings. But even as I'm thinking, *Yeah, baby! Pile it on, pile it on*, the more honest part of me says, *Nope.*

If you and I were dogs, we could bask in that kind of praise with a clear conscience. Dogs can be purely selfless. But human beings have too much "self." Any saint would admit that. Even the best caregivers have moments of being cranky, envious, self-pitying, depressed, anxious, peevish, downright mad, bored, lonely, impatient . . .

Did I leave anything out?

Oh, right. Tired. But that never happens to caregivers. Which reminds me, we need to add "sarcastic" to the list.

Now, here's the real question: Is complete selflessness the right goal for a caregiver?

For the first months after David came home from his lengthy rehabilitation at Denver's Craig Hospital, I *was* selfless. When we showered, I lavished shampoo, time, and energy on him, but I felt guilty giving myself more than the most basic scrubbing. I ate quickly so I could help him with meals. The only doctors I saw were his. Ditto for things like vitamins.

One morning, when I took him in to work, a teammate asked how I was doing. I said, "Fine," and shifted the subject to David's well-being. She laughed. "You remind me of my mom. All she thinks about is my dad."

That bothered me. I stuffed it, but it kept poking me.

A few days later, during a transfer from wheelchair to car, it seemed David was about to whack his head against the door frame. Reaching to protect him, I misjudged and gave him a good slap in the face.

David looked surprised. I burst into tears.

He said jokingly, "You hit me, and *you're* crying?" But I couldn't laugh. As he listened, astonished,

I sobbed out my overwhelming sense of guilt, responsibility, and failure. This moment had been building for a long time, and it was clear to both of us that something had to change.

If you haven't heard some version of "Caregivers have to take care of themselves, or they'll have nothing to give," you will. The staff at Craig Hospital made sure I did. But on discharge day, that wise and necessary principle somehow got lost in the hour-long drive from Denver to our new normal in Colorado Springs. It took several months and a slap in the face—David's face—for me to find it again.

Since then, I've kept it clearly in sight.

"Selfless" sounds a lot better than it really is. Losing yourself isn't good for either you or your person. There's a broad, healthy space between selfish and selfless, and it has plenty of room for both of you.

So, flap those saintly wings. But keep your paws on the ground.

11

THE RIGHT KIND
OF ADDICTION

_____

There's always a light. You just have to turn it on.

MOLLY BURKE, *It's Not What It Looks Like*

WHEN IT COMES TO TAKING CARE of yourself, there's something you need to know. I learned it the hard way.

In your brain, the hypothalamus keeps a firm grip on aspects of life like appetite, sleep, and metabolism. *Hugely* important. But certain behaviors can knock your hypothalamus out of whack and drench it in dopamine. This becomes an addiction. You want to have the feeling again and again, so you do whatever it takes.

That's what happened to me.

Craig Hospital in Denver has a world-wide reputation for their rehab work with spinal-cord injuries. Bit by bit, they got David off the ventilator, up in a wheelchair, and working with therapists. Finally, they moved him from his room next to the nurses' desk—one reserved for a physically unstable patient likely to need immediate help—to a two-room suite at the far end of the hall. This suite, a symbol of his improvement, meant I could stay with him.

All good. Right?

Yes, but . . .

I missed my nightly break from the hospital. No more walking the short distance to my family-housing apartment and curling up in bed with a book, away from the medical sounds, smells, and lack of privacy. David tried to let me sleep through the night, but sometimes he simply couldn't. Nights were especially rough for him, and he wanted me near. He felt anxious, fearful, overwhelmed by the uncertainties of this new life. So did I. He had no break from it, and now I didn't either.

That's when my addiction got started. One night, before I trudged off to my sofa bed in the other half of David's suite, we decided to spend our last few minutes together being thankful. Out loud, intentionally, specifically thankful.

We thanked God for our reliable car. For the night

nurse who massaged David's hands with lotion when he couldn't sleep. Family. Friends. Getting the halo off. Good medical insurance, which had kicked in barely two weeks before the accident . . . for which our insurance company probably felt much less thankful.

The next morning, I rolled out of bed and went into David's room for another dose of thankfulness. This became our pattern. First thing in the morning, last thing at night.

Wow. We had no idea what those few minutes would do.

Our circumstances didn't change, but our attitudes did. Hospital staff began making comments like "I love coming into your room. It's so peaceful." And it was— because *we* were. Not perfect, of course, but much better than I would have thought possible.

Since then, I've learned that thankfulness physically changes your brain. The dopamine it sends to your hypothalamus creates a natural high, and stress hormones can't stand up under that. A single event of thankfulness has a long-lasting effect on your outlook.

And the benefits don't stop there. This natural high brings less pain, deeper sleep, better health, more energy, and lower likelihood of depression.[1] It also creates an addiction to being kind and doing good to other people. Seriously! Exactly what every caregiver needs.

Remember Mrs. Hastings, the tiny woman with joyful eyes? Remember how she smiled and said of her bedbound husband, "I'm so thankful I can have him here with me"?

She definitely had the right kind of addiction.

12

BOXING WITH
THE PROS

We walk away to a smattering of applause from the Lookers.

DANIEL TAYLOR, *Do We Not Bleed?*

WRITING ABOUT THANKFULNESS was a good reminder
for me. It's easy to let the habit slide, to forget what a
good and powerful ally thankfulness can be.

Fatigue, on the other hand, is the neighborhood
bully. When fatigue comes swaggering in, even thankfulness runs for cover. There you stand, all on your own,
feeling heavy, hopeless, and fuzzy-brained. You can't
imagine ever *not* being tired.

Early on, a writer friend read the rough draft of
this book. She got to the tale of David's disastrous late-
night catheter change. "Whoa," she said. "A story about
incontinence? That's kind of jarring." She read it again.

This time, she looked thoughtful. "But I suppose for caregivers, it's reality."

For many of us, that's exactly what it is.

David and I have had plenty of these experiences. A valve left open on his catheter bag, probably by me. A bag that develops a leak. A blow-off of the external catheter itself. The first category usually requires no more than wiping the floor and changing his shoes. The second might include his socks. The third always means a major cleanup.

My patience in this has surprised us both. I've done okay even with category-three events that required as much time and labor as the night of the disaster. Not perfect—my saintly wings still don't get me off the ground—but good. Amazingly good, considering my pre-accident track record of impatience. So, what made that night different?

The neighborhood bully: fatigue.

That night, David and I had stayed up way too late. I was already sagging as we rolled into the bedroom, with at least half an hour of nighttime preps ahead. But at last, I swung his legs up onto the bed, which meant only the catheter change stood between me and my pillow. Off with the old condom catheter, on with the skin prep. As always, I wished the skin prep didn't take so long to dry before the new catheter could go on. I redeemed the time by cleaning the leg bag and hanging it in the shower. Then, night bag in hand, I came out of the bathroom to see—

Disaster. Sleeping man. Catheter not yet on. Even if you've forgotten the story, you can guess what happened.

All this time, I'd been telling myself, *Hang in there. You can do it. Just a few more minutes.* Now the reality of another hour-plus of cleanup, laundry, and putting everything back together hit like a knockout punch.

My hands were fists. Affliction had a choke hold on beauty. My strand in the safety net was unraveling fast. And nothing about my reaction could be called either heroic or quiet. "I don't believe it!" I shouted, leaping around the room. "How could you *do* this to me?"

I wanted to die. Literally. At least then I could sleep.

That was my tipping point. Yours might not be incontinence, but you have something. Something that howls, *Too much! I can't do this.* Every caregiver has something like that. And that's why David asked me to put this story in the book. He said he didn't mind a little embarrassment for himself.

"I know how being tired drains all the life out of

you," he told me. "I watched you struggle that night and heard you say, 'I can't do this.' But then I saw you make the choice to start doing it. And I thought, *She's getting stronger.*"

The neighborhood bully looms over us, boxing gloves raised, sneering, "Give up. This is too hard for a wimp like you." But he's almost always wrong, and David is right. Each time we push ourselves to our feet to face the bully again, we become a little stronger.

13

DIVIDE AND CONQUER

And for tired eyes every light is too bright,
and for tired lips every breath too heavy,
and for tired ears every word too much.

GEORG BÜCHNER, *Leonce and Lena*

WHICH DO YOU PICTURE MORE CLEARLY?

A car . . . or a blue Honda Civic.

A dog . . . or a young, high-spirited Irish Setter.

A person . . . or a middle-aged woman with a nose ring and fading tattoos.

Some categories are just too big and generic to get a grip on. That's true for me, anyway. Dividing them into smaller, detailed pieces gives a chance to step back and really *see* them. That happened recently when David was listening to his Audible Audiobooks account and called me over to join him. "I think you'll like this," he said and punched the play button.

A deep voice rolled out. "The alternative to soul-acceptance is soul-fatigue."[1]

Fatigue again. Hadn't I had enough of that? But the narrator went on to tackle the bully in a way I hadn't thought about before.

"There is a kind of fatigue," he said, "that attacks the body."

He gave examples. Staying up too late, like the night of our disastrous catheter change. Compensating for shortage of sleep with coffee in the morning and an energy drink in the afternoon. Not exercising. Eating unhealthy foods.

Not much new there, but then he said, "There is a kind of fatigue that attacks the mind."

Information overload. Screens everywhere. Carrying around "mental lists of errands not yet done and bills not yet paid and emails not yet replied to." Trying to stuff our negative emotions, "like holding beach balls under the water." All this, he said, makes the mind grow weary.

Then he talked about "a kind of fatigue that attacks the will."

So many choices. So many decisions. And so many of them we're not qualified to make. How do we know when to say yes and when to say no? Sometimes we just say yes to everything because our will is too worn out to choose.

The neighborhood bully looks crushingly big. But what happens if we divide him up like this? If we can identify which part dumps the most weight on us— fatigue of body, mind, or will—maybe we can do something about it. Divide and conquer.

In the past, I would have said, "This is great! I need to read the whole book." David got a lot out of it, and so did I from hearing just that one small section. I'd like to know more about soul-acceptance, since the author calls it an alternative to soul-fatigue. It sounds hopeful.

But "books not yet read" fits into his description of mental lists and mind fatigue. So, yes, I'd like to read it. But I don't have to. Maybe I learned all I needed to from that book, at least for now. Maybe now is the time to use what I already learned.

Is it my imagination, or did the bully just shrink a little?

Now he might even fit into that blue Honda Civic with the young, high-spirited Irish Setter and the middle-aged woman with a nose ring and faded tattoos.

14

WELL-KEPT

We ourselves feel that what we are
doing is just a drop in the ocean.

MOTHER TERESA

BY THE TIME WE FOUND A PARKING SPOT, David and I were running late for his appointment at the VA hospital. As we headed for the building, with me propelling his manual wheelchair at warp speed, we passed a group of veterans hanging around outside the entrance. Most sat in wheelchairs.

One man called, "How ya doin'?"

David said hi. I smiled but kept us moving. We didn't want to lose this appointment. When the automatic doors opened to let us in, I heard the man say approvingly to those around him, "He looks well-kept."

I laughed. Then I stopped laughing. The man who

had spoken obviously *wasn't* well-kept. None of those men looked good. Baggy clothes that didn't seem quite clean. Scruffy beards. Shaggy, greasy hair. Why were they hanging around the parking lot like that? Waiting for one of those services that provides a ride for people in wheelchairs? Useful, but you do have to wait.

Without the safety net of my care, that could be David. Unkempt, uncared for. Vulnerable.

Without your care, that could be *your* person.

What do you tell yourself about your work as a caregiver? Does the tedium of so much you have to do beat you down sometimes? Cleaning the catheter bag with vinegar water every morning and evening, staring off into space as you shake the bag up and down, side to side. Sorting meds into the weekly pillbox. Driving your person to medical appointments, searching for a parking spot, then hustling into the office to fill out forms and wait. Laundry. Meals. Cleanup. Getting your person pajamaed and into bed at night, showered and dressed in the morning. And let's not even mention that devilish invention, compression socks.

If that made you laugh, you know what I'm talking about.

For a lot of us, it isn't just the repetitious nature of

those tasks. It's the smallness. David and I have a friend who runs a huge homeless shelter. He serves five hundred people every night and has wild stories to tell. Another friend volunteers for a city charity I strongly believe in. I'd like to be part of that big work, but I can't commit with any consistency. My commitment is to one person.

One person. How small that sounds. How insignificant.

"We ourselves feel that what we are doing is just a drop in the ocean." Mother Teresa, whose lifelong work with the neediest of humanity won a Nobel Peace Prize, said this to a friend. Then she added, "But if that drop was not there, I think the ocean would be less by that missing drop. We don't have to think in numbers. We can only love one person at a time—serve one person at a time."[1]

One person.

Your person is clean and cared for, because you gave yourself to that work today. Your person doesn't have to wait in the parking lot, because you're there with the car. All those small, tedious tasks you do weave together to keep your safety net of care strong and in good condition.

Well-kept.

15

THE IDEA MAN HITS
A HOME RUN

_____

Carry each other's burdens.
GALATIANS 6:2, NIV

DAVID ALWAYS HAS LOTS OF IDEAS. Some I like, some not so much. Historically, the ones I've liked least have turned out to be the best.

When he decided to sign up with a home health care agency, I resisted. Strongly! I'd been his only caregiver for almost two years. I couldn't imagine having a stranger in our home, doing what I'm supposed to do.

But he held firm. "You need a morning off," he said. "Just once a week. And then if you got sick and couldn't take care of me for a few days, we would already have the connection. They'd send someone to help me."

A backup safety net? That made sense.

So, we signed up. Since then, we've had a wild variety of certified nursing assistants (CNAs) come through our home, and we've learned which qualities are essential for us. Commitment to David's safety, of course, and willingness to fit into our ways. Punctuality— important because David has a job to get to—has proved a common problem. After two years with one otherwise-terrific CNA who was leaving the agency, we knew to turn down a possible replacement when she warned us, "I'm not a morning person. I have trouble being on time."

Beautiful honesty. A large, slow-moving woman, she wouldn't have fit well into our tight schedule or equally tight quarters.

What we didn't expect was how far above "acceptable" most of these CNAs would rise. They became part of our household, trusted friends with their own dreams and worries. Each time we heard that our helper was moving away or taking a different job, we mourned. "We'll never have anyone as good," we told each other.

But almost without exception, the next one was as good or better. I wish you could meet Beth, who was our CNA when I first wrote this. She's a treat. She now copes with scheduling for the agency, which is a tough job. Then came Antoinette, who handled David with strength and tenderness, loved our super-sweet coffee, and made us laugh. She moved out of state.

This brings up the big issue.

In ten years, we've gone through well over a dozen CNAs. And, no, it isn't just us. Turnover is an industry-wide problem. Most of the ones who left us wanted to stay in the job but couldn't afford to. They simply didn't make a living wage.

This is just *wrong*. These CNAs, mostly young women, drive their own cars long distances through all kinds of weather, in daylight and darkness, to take care of strangers. Several have told us they consider this a privilege. None have ever spoken to David with anger or made him feel ashamed. Instead, we've experienced their hard work, integrity, cheerfulness, strength, intelligence, determination, self-sacrifice, kindness. I could fill pages.

I wish I could also fill their bank accounts. They deserve it.

If you're already using home health care, I hope your experience has been as good as ours. If you're considering it, I can attest that this was one of David's best ideas. I never imagined what that regular morning break would do for me.

And if you're one of the CNAs, thank you. You are God's blessing to those who most need it.

What does your home health care certified nursing assistant (CNA) want from you?

1. A routine they can fit into.

2. Supplies kept organized and stocked.

3. "Please," "thanks," and being listened to. If your person acts like a demanding grouch with the CNA, your attitude can soften that.

4. Not expected, but nice: a periodic cash gift. Let them know it's not a tip, which they have to report, but a thank-you gift.

16

THE SECOND
ELEPHANT

Between us and heaven or hell there is only life,
which is the most fragile thing in the world.

BLAISE PASCAL, _Pensées_

REMEMBER THE ELEPHANT IN THE ROOM? Big and
pushy, he lurks behind every caregiver, muttering, _What
if I can't do this? What if I fail?_

I hope this book helps you shove that elephant
against the wall. He might never leave completely, but
at least you won't have him blocking your light. You
could even put him to work. Hang towels to dry on his
tusks, or train him to clear out high cobwebs with his
clever, pliable trunk.

But many caregivers have a second elephant crowd-
ing the room, and this one definitely won't go away.

My person could die any time. How do I live with that?

This question came from a friend whose husband has cancer. I asked other caregivers for their ideas but didn't get far. Most of those in my friend's position didn't want to think about the topic. Others asked me to come back when I got answers because they wanted to know too. Caregivers whose person had died recently felt too raw to open themselves to the question, and those with more time to grieve had lost the immediacy of their emotions.

That left me on my own. David has a disability rather than a progressive disease, but the nature of his injury has taken him to the edge a number of times. I'll probably outlive him. I hope I do because he needs my care. At the same time, I don't *want* him to die before me.

Those are the kinds of thoughts that go around and around. Sound familiar? I've gone that circular route many times. This time, though, my friend's question took me in an unexpected direction.

Blaise Pascal was a French mathematician, physicist, inventor, writer, and Catholic theologian in the 1600s, a brilliant man. I first heard him quoted years ago, and the words stayed with me: "Between us and heaven or hell there is only life, which is the most fragile thing in the world."

People have written books about the first half of that. But the last part is what stands out to me now. Is life really "the most fragile thing in the world"?

Human beings can be amazingly tough. Think of all the people you've heard of who should have died but didn't. Nurses in the critical care unit called David "the miracle man" because breaking his neck on that bike path should have killed him. But he's still alive.

Then I remember friends of ours who have died in the years since his accident. They were healthy and whole when David lay breathing through a ventilator in the hospital, but now they're gone. All sorts of causes: quick, slow, violent, natural. Anyone can die at any time, including you or me.

When David and I got married, our best man arrived from overseas the evening before the wedding and had to leave right after. David hadn't seen Mike in years. They were both in the military but had never been stationed near each other, and I'd never even heard of him. I didn't ask why David chose him for that honor, but I wondered.

A few months after the wedding, Mike was killed in a flying accident.

"I almost didn't ask him to be best man," David

told me then, "but I knew he wouldn't come all that way otherwise. We had a long talk the morning of the wedding. It's so good we got that last time together. We really reconnected, and I knew Mike was doing okay."

If life *is* the most fragile thing of all, what do we do with that? Get scared and depressed? I'm no stranger to those emotions and could easily go that way, spending my days in the shadow of the second elephant. Instead, I want to do what I saw David choose with Mike.

I want to treasure the time.

17

CLIMB IN THE CAR

You're short on ears and long on mouth.

JOHN WAYNE'S character in *Big Jake*

"YOU'RE A *TERRIBLE* LISTENER," I SAID.

That was no more and no less than the truth. This guy rarely made good eye contact. Anyone talking to him got maybe half of his attention. The rest of his mind was busy putting together his own reply, or off on some unrelated subject.

This time, though, I got his total, astonished focus. And what a good thing! My husband took my long-ago words so seriously—did you guess that's who I was talking about?—he's now a counselor and one of the best listeners I know. Now he teaches *me* how to listen well.

Actually, we're both still learning. It's a lifelong process.

In Bekah DiFelice's lovely nonfiction book, *Almost There*, an acquaintance tells Bekah that she used to think people shared part of their story because they wanted her to do the same. Then she realized that wasn't so. "People need to process out loud and have the space to do it," she says. "They don't want someone to hijack their story by telling theirs. So now I try to simply listen."[1]

I love that term, *hijack*. It's so expressive. And its opposite makes me think of choosing to climb in the passenger side and ride along while the other person drives. Choosing to "simply listen."

For the last seven years of her life, my mother lived with my sister and brother-in-law. When Jann and Steve took some days away for the birth of their first grandchild, I stayed with Mom. She'd been depressed for a while, which was unusual for her. During my stay, she mostly wanted to sleep instead of talk, so I honored that.

It's one of my deep regrets. I wish I'd tried to draw her out, to ask questions and really listen. She probably needed that then more than any other time. Mom lived another five years and got plenty of enjoyment out of them, largely thanks to the good and loving care

Jann and Steve gave her. But I'd wasted an important opportunity.

Listen, listen, listen.

David has plenty of people who care about what he says. But I'm in a special category, and he tells me things he wouldn't tell anyone else. I need to listen well. You may be in the same position. Or maybe your person is more isolated, and you're the only listener they have. Or maybe your person can't physically communicate.

Whatever your situation, I hope you have someone who listens well to *you*. My friend Sharon loves her caregiver support group. Another caregiver I know ditched her own group, because too much hijacking and too little listening left her empty. Instead, she gets together with a couple of friends who know what she needs.

They climb in the car with her and "simply listen."

I wish for you at least one person who listens well. Looking for a caregiver support group? Your primary-care physician can point you to some. Also, Stephen Ministry trains people in a church to "listen to, care for, and walk with those going through difficult times in life."[2] Someone will come to your house if you want.

18

GOING DOWN

---

*Love in practice is a harsh and dreadful thing
compared to love in dreams.*

FYODOR DOSTOYEVSKY,
The Brothers Karamazov

SIX TALL STEPS OF BRICK AND concrete connect our
porch to the front sidewalk. Their steepness explains
why we couldn't build our wheelchair ramp there. To
meet slope requirement codes, any ramp going down
those front steps would have to end halfway across the
street.

One morning, when David and I sat on the front
porch having coffee, I got up to go into the house for
refills. As I reached for his cup, he said, "Don't leave me
out here alone."

I laughed.

He didn't. "I don't feel safe," he said. "Those steps . . ."

A man we'd met at Craig Hospital popped into my mind. After years as a paraplegic, Jack had accidentally tipped his wheelchair down a flight of stairs and become a quad. His lack of bitterness and warm encouragement of other patients put him high on my list of quiet heroes. But the thought of that crippling plunge always made me feel shivery. Maybe David had been thinking of him too.

"Are you afraid you might fall down the steps?" I asked. "You're nowhere near them. Just stay where you are."

"I'm not afraid of falling. I'm afraid I'll do it on purpose."

Life stopped. The background noises of traffic went mute. I put down both cups and sat.

We talked. The previous year, scar tissue in David's neck had decreased his mobility and ramped up his nerve pain. Surgery stopped the downward trend, with a fifty percent chance of getting him back to his version of normal. We'd strongly hoped for that. But it hadn't happened.

Without that hope, he told me now, the pain seemed unendurable. The idea of suicide had sneaked in . . . and stayed. "I never looked for an opportunity," he said.

"But the thought keeps getting more intense. I've been ashamed to tell you, but I knew I had to. I was afraid sometime when you weren't out here with me, I'd just roll over to the steps and do it."

I'd had no idea. I wouldn't have even thought to ask.

For David, this time on the porch marked a turning point. Being taken seriously, really listened to, drained the power out of those thoughts. He no longer felt alone. He decided he didn't need professional help—a counselor himself, he could meet with someone on our team for that. But he promised to tell me if any suicidal ideation showed up again. Even the faintest breath of it.

I believe him. But whenever he seems a little off, I check in. It's scary to do that. I have to brace myself to ask, then stay with it and encourage him to talk about what's going on.

Lately, more and more of our medical appointments include a short mental-health survey that asks about suicidal thoughts. The VA has done that for a while because of veteran trauma, but now I see it everywhere. I like it. Filling out the form together gives me a natural way to check in.

Five things David wants you to know:

1. When I first came home from
    the hospital and thought I would
    never have a life again, I hid in
    sleep. Long naps, two or three
    times a day. The opposite—
    having trouble sleeping—can
    also mean depression. If your
    person loses their appetite
    or their usual interests, that's
    a heads-up too.

2. Talking about this is vital. Be
    direct.

3. If they express negative feelings
    to you, listen. Don't try to talk
    them out of those feelings.

4. If they pull in and isolate them-
    selves, ask. Sometimes when my
    pain is high, I don't want to be a

burden to Jill, so I get quiet. But I've learned that my silence is the heaviest burden I can lay on her.

5. Pain and hopelessness aren't logical. That idea of throwing myself and my wheelchair down the porch steps . . . not smart. Most likely, I would have ended up with a lot *more* pain and hopelessness. So don't dismiss what you notice just because it doesn't make sense.

19

TIME FOR A TWEAK

Variety's the very spice of life,
that gives it all its flavour.

WILLIAM COWPER, *The Task*

WHY DID I FEEL SO BLAH AFTER EVERY MEAL?

I've never been a terrific cook, but the problem had nothing to do with the food. This was more a sense of not connecting with David while we ate. We always talked, but the time together left me feeling flat. Lonely.

During dinner one night, I finally told him how I felt.

"Maybe we should change where you sit," he said. "It's hard for me to turn my head and look at you. Try sitting straight across from me."

We were seated at right angles, with me at the short end of the table and to his left. We'd established that pattern when we first came home from Craig Hospital, since it let me feed both myself and him. But we didn't need that anymore. Thanks to time, therapy, and self-discipline, he could now manage meals on his own.

What he couldn't do was turn his head far to the left. He had more range of motion to the right, but straight ahead worked best. I shifted myself and my dinner, picked up my spoon, and looked across the table at David.

Instant eye contact. We both smiled. Instant connection.

How simple! And how amazingly effective.

In our months at Craig Hospital, the staff had given me a good grounding in how to be David's caregiver. Our last week there, they had me do all his care so going home wouldn't come as such a shock. I tried to do everything exactly as the CNAs there did.

"You'll tweak a lot of this after you've been home awhile," one nurse said. "You'll figure out what works best for the two of you."

She was right. In those first months home, we did a lot of tweaking. But as we talked that night at dinner, we realized this counted as our first tweak in quite a while. We'd stopped actively looking for areas that could use a change. So, what else had become a blind spot? I studied him critically. Maybe those easy-to-pull-on black sweatpants looked a little too casual for being back at work.

We decided to add "monthly evaluation" to the schedule.

Oh, great, you're probably thinking. *Here's another thing I ought to do.*

No. No, no, no, and definitely no. The last thing I want to do is add pressure. Do you think David and I actually *do* the evaluation every month? No.

But just seeing those words on the calendar sometimes jogs my brain into action. Sometimes we come up with a way for David to do a task I've been doing for him, which encourages both of us. Sometimes he's moved backward in some area, and our longstanding routine doesn't work as well anymore. That's discouraging but necessary to acknowledge. So, we tweak the routine.

Plenty of times, we then have to tweak the tweak, but that's okay. You can't expect them all to be as elegantly simple as "Try sitting straight across from me."

That was a good one!

20

MELTDOWN AT THE AUTO SUPPLY STORE

The more choices you have . . .
the less you're going to feel like a victim.

DR. EDITH EVA EGER, *The Choice*

THE FIRST SUMMER AFTER DAVID'S ACCIDENT, I tried to replace a headlight bulb in our Chevy. Did you know some cars have two separate bulbs on each side, one for high beam and one for low, located in different places, with one hiding behind the other?

I didn't. Not until I went back to the auto supply store, frustrated and sweaty, to report that no amount of contorting myself under the car's hood would make the bulb fit.

Oh, the contempt in that salesman's face and voice . . .

As they say in novels, something snapped. I didn't exactly shout, but everyone in the store heard me tell him, "My husband is a quadriplegic, I'm trying to make life work, and *you* aren't helping!" Then I flung myself away from the sales desk and headed for the door.

"Hey," he called after me. "You didn't get your refund."

"I don't *want* my refund!" I sounded about two years old.

Outdoors, I melted against the car and sobbed. Another salesman hurried out to apologize. He ended by installing the right bulb in the right place while I sniffed and hiccupped behind him. Then I drove away in deep humiliation. I had never made a scene like that before and hope I never do again. I can't go back to that store.

Here's the good part: I don't have to. David and I crossed "auto maintenance" off my list. I now put gas in the car and take it to Jiffy Lube once a year to have them change the oil, but that's all. That's enough.

Depending on your person's situation, you're dealing with doctors, nurses, CNAs, physical therapists, occupational therapists, dietitians, CPAP providers, pharmacists, and people with other medical occupations you can't even pronounce. You come home from each appointment and try to do everything they told you. And let's not forget all the regular demands like cleaning, cooking, laundry, and grocery shopping, not to mention dealing with bills and insurance.

Right. Let's *not* mention that.

Maybe you also have young children. Or maybe you're among those who work an outside job, then come home and dive straight into caregiving. Or maybe you have young children *and* a job. If so, I don't know how you do it. Because we can't do it all.

Each medical specialist seems to believe theirs is the only field, or at least the most essential. As she straps your person into the standing frame, the therapist says to you, "Last week, I gave you a daily list of passive range exercises to do for her arms and legs. Morning and evening, one hour for each session. How'd that go?"

"Great," you say. "I think it's helping."

"You did the exercises every day?"

"Five days," you say. "Well—" a burst of honesty "—four and a half."

She slides you a long, cool look. "Only nine sessions? For the whole week?"

Implied: *You slacker*. And for that moment, you feel like a failure. You're ashamed. You know the exercises are important for your person.

But so is everything else.

If science ever decides to clone people, they should start with caregivers. But until that happens, we'll just have to focus on the must-dos and call it good. The should-dos can go in a drawer, out of sight but available when priorities change.

If you're thinking that's easy to say but hard to do, you're in good company. We *want* to do it all. But we can't. For me, the drawer visual helps. Tucking the should-dos into that drawer means I don't have to wade through them to get to the must-dos. If for some reason I pull one out and do something with it, that's a bonus.

As for the sense of failure and shame that wants to drag along behind us, we can roll that up with all the don't-dos—tasks like auto maintenance—and shove them under the bed. Not only does that get them out of sight, but we have a great excuse not to vacuum under there.

21

THE THIRD ELEPHANT

I'm better. Thanks for asking. Not cured of course.
What would that mean anyway? Cured of the human condition?

DANIEL TAYLOR, *Do We Not Bleed?*

FIRST ELEPHANT. *What if I can't do this? What if I fail?*

Second elephant. *My person could die any time. How do I live with that?*

Now meet the third elephant. He isn't actually in the room. Instead, he lurks just outside the door, immense and shadowy, swaying from side to side and whispering. His words are quiet but distinct.

Sometimes I wish my person would *die.*

Nell Noonan wrote an honest little book called *The Struggles of Caregiving: 28 Days of Prayer*. In one chapter, she tells about a woman in her Alzheimer's support group who feels trapped by her husband's illness.

Though the wife knows he can't help the way he behaves, she gets angry with him and then feels terrible. Another member agonizes because he can no longer remember what his wife was like "before." He'd never thought this could happen, and he feels guilty and ashamed.

Noonan herself has times of anger and desperation that she calls her "widow wish."

Her honesty comes in part from comments readers made about her earlier book, *Not Alone: Encouragement for Caregivers*. Some told her it "did not go deep enough into guilt and dark thoughts."[1] One woman wrote that she sometimes wished her mother would die and be finished with the misery of this life. She asked if thinking that way was wrong.

Noonan gave a good answer, which you'll get if you read her book. But for now, here's my opinion: Right, wrong, or neutral, that kind of thinking is bound to push its way out sometimes. And letting it come into the light is the healthiest thing we can do.

A few years before David's accident, our family went through a hard, scary time. Dread of what might happen clawed at the back door of my mind. The more I tried to keep it shut away in darkness, the deeper the claws gouged. Finally, I gave up.

"All right," I said aloud. "What's the absolute worst that could happen?"

Having opened that door, I waited to see what came. It was bad. But instead of collapsing in despair, I had a sense of relief. What came marching through the door didn't surprise me. I'd known about it all this time, but pretending it didn't exist had wasted energy and made the claws seem bigger and sharper than they really were. I felt stronger. Even if the worst happened, God would still be *with me*.

On paper, that just looks like words. But its reality filled my soul. I'd faced the worst, and it had no power.

Some things I have to learn many times. Not this one. As soon as I catch myself trying to hold that door shut, I step back and let it swing wide open. Think the thought. Look at it up close. Out in the light, it usually proves more reasonable than I'd expected.

So, am I saying that to wish your person would die is reasonable?

Yes. For a lot of caregivers, the third elephant makes perfect sense. If our person is in mental or physical misery, it's natural to wish they could be free. Any threads of selfishness in this wish shouldn't surprise us either. We're human, and caregiving is hard. For Noonan, acknowledging her "widow wish" has kept darkness from giving it more power than it should hold.

So, bring that elephant into the room. Let him join the other two.

He's much smaller than you thought.

22

IT CAN HAPPEN

_____

Poppies. Poppies. Poppies will put them to sleep.
Sle-ee-p. Now they'll sle-ee-p . . .

WICKED WITCH OF THE WEST IN
The Wizard of Oz

CLEARLY, SO CLEARLY, I see my forefinger and thumb putting one pill into David's mouth, then the second one. I slip the straw between his lips. He swallows. And so begins the slide toward death.

Not a nightmare. Not murder. Not assisted suicide. Accident.

Five years ago, I gave David an accidental overdose. The meds were exactly what the ER doctor had prescribed and sent home with us the night before. One oxycodone and one Valium. The combination wouldn't have overdosed most people, but it proved too much for someone in David's compromised physical state. He sank deeply into sleep.

At first, I didn't worry. I knew he was exhausted from the pain of yet another compression fracture, followed by a five-hour wait at the ER that went late into the night. And now, I'd just given him his morning dose of painkillers. I *expected* him to sleep deeply. I thought it would be good for him.

Fatigue had a heavy grip on me too. I felt dazed, my judgment blurry. It took several hours for me to realize this snoring sleep of his wasn't normal.

When I tried to wake him but got no response, I called a nurse friend. She told me to get in David's face and shout his name. "If that doesn't work," she said, "push hard on his chest and keep shouting. Do that until he wakes up."

But he didn't wake up. He'd gone way too deep for that.

"Okay," she said. "It's time to call 911."

The twelve years since David's bicycle accident have been a gift. These last five are a double gift. If he had died from the overdose, how could I bear the image of my hand giving him those two pills? Instead, he lost only a day. I lived that day for both of us, and it just about did me in.

We learned a few things.

The paramedics who came to our house gave David naloxone, which reverses the effects of an opioid. It can save someone whose breathing has slowed or even stopped recently. If your person ever takes opioids—things like oxycodone, hydrocodone, fentanyl, Percocet—it's good to have naloxone around. In most states, you can buy this without a prescription.[1]

Once the naloxone had taken hold, the paramedic said, "Now it's just the Valium talking." Valium isn't an opioid. It's a benzodiazepine, or "benzo," and has nothing like naloxone to counteract it. With David as stable as they could make him, the paramedics took him to the ER.

There, after what seemed forever, a doctor came into my private waiting room —once again, the kind of room reserved for people with hard news to hear. He said, "We've done all we can. Now it's up to David to declare himself."

A lot of factors came together that morning.

The combination of meds. A flu epidemic that

had last night's ER overwhelmed. Our CNA's asthma attack (we decided to let David sleep while she left to get a treatment, planning to come back later). And, of course, the neighborhood bully who always hangs around after a night like ours. Warning flags popped up several times that morning, but fatigue tucked me under his arm like a football and outran them all.

This kind of perfect storm can happen. You probably know that from experience.

Here's my takeaway: If possible, no more opioids or Valium for David—and definitely not together. If a doctor prescribes one, I intend to ask questions. And I'll be ready to say no.

For now, I'm deeply thankful that David "declared himself," climbing up that long, slow slope into life. I don't have to live with the image of my hands—God's hands, the hands of a caregiver—undoing all these years of careful, loving work in one fuzzy-brained morning of poor judgment.

It can happen.

In the United States, doctors prescribe opioids heavily. Odds of dying from accidental opioid overdose now surpass those of dying in a car accident.[2] And 16 percent of fatal opioid overdoses also involve benzos.[3] The benzo Valium hit David extra hard because one of his daily meds is a benzo as well.

23

BEAUTY INTO UGLINESS

Sticks and stones may break my bones,
but words will rip my skin apart.
ANONYMOUS

DAVID'S DAD STOOD ON ONE SIDE OF HIM. Eddie, our physical-therapist friend, held David's other arm. As they made their slow way down our hall, another friend, Nabeel, followed close behind with a kitchen chair for when David wore out.

I'll never forget the beauty of those moments. Seeing my husband walk for the first time since his accident made *my* legs go weak. The mix of joyful emotions served up a powerful brew. Those three faithful, loving, committed men . . . David's weakness and his determination . . . hope on the move.

Before long, he could do standing transfers. We gave

away our mechanical lift and banished the transfer slide boards to the closet. David especially reveled in getting rid of the temporary ramp in our front yard. We'd rented it by the month, and frugality motivated him to conquer the three steps to our back door before the next payment came due. As time went on, we strolled side by side along the quiet road that winds through our organization's property. Pine trees, birdsong, soft breezes, with the occasional turkey or bighorn sheep wandering past.

True story—all of this really happened. But that last bit didn't look as idyllic as I've made it sound.

David was walking, yes, but not far and not well. During each outing, I helped him stand from his wheelchair, handed him his cane, and watched him take the first slow steps. Then I moved to support his weaker left side. As he walked, he leaned heavily on the cane in his right hand and even more heavily on me. By the time we got back in the car to drive home, my arm and shoulder ached.

As for David, those "strolls" represented a huge effort. With massive self-discipline, he forced himself to walk a little farther each time. But as the months went on, his upper body still bent sharply forward, pulling down against my arm. He could raise his right foot enough to clear the road, but his left shoe scraped.

After that first exciting year, David's progress had leveled out. No matter how hard he worked, he stayed stuck in place.

And now we had a deadline. We'd learned that almost all improvement would happen within the first two and a half years after his accident. That's the nature of nerve damage. Then the window of opportunity would slam shut, and what he had was all he would ever have.

I wanted straight posture and a strong stride. From the glorious, flashing joy of that first walk down the hallway, my attitude had degenerated into anxious dissatisfaction. "Is that the best you can do?" I'd say. "Can't you stand up straighter? You've *got* to lift your feet higher, and you can't when you're bent like that."

The closer we got to the deadline, the more I pushed. I actually said, "You're not *trying*!"

That was too much for David. "Jill, I *am* trying. What you're saying doesn't help."

"Fine," I shot back. "I just won't say anything."

For a couple of days, any walking took place in grim silence. Then one afternoon, without my intending it, a word popped out.

If you want to know, keep reading.

I hope you do. Because this ugly little story needs redemption.

24

REDEEMING THE UGLINESS

Words kill, words give life;
they're either poison or fruit—you choose.

PROVERBS 18:21

LEANING ON HIS CANE, David started down the hall. He paused and straightened slightly.

"Good!" The word popped out of my mouth, surprising us both. His eyes brightened, and his head came up a little higher.

None of my pushing and faultfinding had ever accomplished that.

Catch someone doing something right, and praise them. I'd heard that principle many times. So why did I keep pointing out David's failures? Picking at him. Nagging. Scolding.

I knew exactly why. I was afraid.

If you're like me, your worst life strategies have fear's sweaty fingerprints all over them. With David's window of opportunity only months from slamming shut, he was nowhere near where I wanted him. Not even headed in the right direction. The more fear squeezed me, the more my anger squirted out at him. And the more ineffective that proved, the more I did it.

Fear-driven strategies tend to wear earplugs and blindfolds. When David told me "What you're saying doesn't help," I blocked out the truth of his words. And when I saw how he had to struggle against *my* words just to keep going, I blocked that out too.

In my determination to propel David forward, I'd been shoving him down. Now I watched that one spontaneous "Good!" literally lift him up.

Anger is a guardian emotion. Some emotions, like fear or shame, make us feel wimpy, helpless, vulnerable. But anger feels strong. So, when anger invites itself in to stand guard over those "weak" emotions, covering and protecting them, it's tempting to say, "Wow—thanks. Stay as long as you like."

That's a bad idea. For one thing, it becomes hard to deal with what's really going on inside us because we can't get past the guardian.

For another, anger destroys. Unlike words of encouragement, anger has no power to build hope in either us or our person.

I still stumble in this, and I probably always will. In this area, my saintly wings are especially tattered. But now I'm quicker to see and hear what's going on, and that helps. Awareness always helps. If life feels scary, I know to keep an eye out for anger. And if I feel anger churning, I know to check underneath for fear.

I wish my caregiving experience didn't include this ugly story. But telling it opens a way to redeem its ugliness because a lot of caregivers are right here with me. We all have scary things to deal with. We want to be strong, but we feel weak. Without waiting for an invitation, anger rolls in as a coping strategy and makes itself at home.

Unless something wakes us up to what we're doing—like my experience with David in the hallway—anger can become a permanent part of our caregiving. If my story gives that wake-up call to just one caregiver, that's redemption enough.

25

RUMPELSTILTSKIN GETS IT RIGHT

Color is one of the great things in the world that makes life worth living.

GEORGIA O'KEEFFE

MY FRIEND SHARON WROTE in a recent email, "I've become so overwhelmed with my have-to, need-to, and want-to activities that I can't keep things straight. Part of my stress comes from having things fall through the cracks and then beating myself up for not taking care of my responsibilities."

Can you relate? I can.

Sharon has never liked living by lists. But as she began adapting to life with a husband in the early stages of Alzheimer's, Sharon realized she could either initiate changes or end up buried underneath them. She prefers the first option. "I am finally writing down ALL my chores and at least having them recorded in one place, so I can make conscious decisions about my priorities for the day."

Now comes the part I really like.

"Interestingly, the spark that got me started was deciding that my list would be recorded in a small and lovely little journal that I can safely tuck into my hand-bag and keep readily available. I had been saving my cherished journal for something really special. I love holding this little faux-suede book in my hands and delighting in the sumptuous feel of it. The soft cover is black, and the page edges are tinted with rainbow colors. My favorite part of it, though, is the Georgia O'Keeffe quote engraved on the front cover: 'Color is one of the great things in the world that makes life worth living.' I look forward to holding the journal, and that inspires me to keep tabs on things and create a bit of order in my life."

Beauty again. It keeps showing up. But instead of piercing the human heart, this kind of beauty comforts us.

I know because I have something like that. Mine is a tissue box I bought the week after David came home from Craig Hospital. Of unfinished wood, it begged for the creative touch. I set it on the far end of our kitchen counter along with a paintbrush, a jar of water, and tiny bottles of acrylic paint.

In my free moments, which often *were* literally just moments, I penciled a design on the box and painted it. Bit by bit, the box came to colorful life. It took more than a month, but that was okay. I needed the process more than the product.

Dipping my brush into the rich ooze of color and stroking it onto the wood did something important for me. I'd guess the same is true for Sharon as she holds the warm texture of her journal, opens it, and sees the colors ripple by. She isn't just putting up with an unwanted necessity. She's shaping it to enrich her life. Like Rumpelstiltskin in the old fairy tale, she's weaving straw into gold.

That's hopeful. If a to-do list can become a thing of beauty, anything is possible.

26

THE ROAD OF
SABBATICAL RHYTHM

Hello, lamppost, what'cha knowin'?
I've come to watch your flowers growin'.

PAUL SIMON, "The 59th Street Bridge Song (Feelin' Groovy)"

IT'S BETTER TO BURN OUT THAN RUST OUT. Ever heard that before?

Like most adages, this one is clever and catchy—and incomplete. Since when did burning out or rusting out become our only two choices? Or, as a friend of ours said, "Can God count to three?"

Extremes are like ditches. We can travel in one or the other, but the road running along between them has more elbow room and a better view.

David and I serve on the member care team of the organization we work for. Twice a year, our team puts on a seminar to help staff going on sabbatical get ready to use the time well. I love this seminar. It's so useful, people from other organizations come as well.

Some time ago, our organization figured out that people who take a sabbatical every seven to ten years do better in the long run. They stay healthier. They can keep going. If they're on track for burnout, the break lets them rest. It also gives them a chance to consider *why* they're burning out and make some changes.

David and I joined our member care team in June 2009. Two months later, he took a six-month sabbatical . . . though everyone says breaking his neck and being in the hospital doesn't count for that. Either way, we came due again a few years ago. But we didn't take one.

Instead, because of his limitations, we try to live what we call a "sabbatical rhythm of life." That could be the smartest decision we ever made, except it isn't, because we didn't *decide* to do this. We more slid into it. When we overdid, we paid for that. When we built in margin, we had more energy. When we said yes to everything, we got stressed. When we said no to a few things, oh, glorious peace. We stayed healthier. We could keep going.

David and I might be slow learners, but we finally caught on. Those principles we'd helped other people use actually work! So, here's a glimpse of what a sabbatical rhythm of life looks like for us.

- We're outdoors as much as possible. When the weather cooperates, I spend time among the flowers before getting David up in the morning. Our coffee tastes better out there too.

- Instead of movies or TV, we have books. A book goes at your own pace and doesn't make noise. As well as what we're reading individually, we keep a mutual read-aloud going, a chapter each evening—two or three if it's exciting.

- During the week, we try to have only one evening commitment, with Saturdays totally free. That's especially good just before or after a demanding season.

- If something extra jams its way in, we drop something else. We'll have takeout pizza instead of cooking or skip an event where we won't be missed.

- We try to allow more time to get ready for something than we think we need, especially if it involves going somewhere. This is a weak link, but we keep working on it.

This way of life keeps our muscles toned for when hard things, like a night at the ER, throw us into a pothole. Because they will—they do. But it's easier to climb out when you aren't already exhausted.

Can God count to three?

Yes! And so can we.

27

IT IS WHAT IT IS

_____

In this world you will have trouble.

JOHN 16:33, NIV

"WHAT HAPPENED?" David asked.

The man across from us set down his knife and fork. "Oh, some guy broke into my house one night when I was in bed. I heard a noise and went out in the hall." He touched his bruised face. "I don't remember anything after that."

"That's terrible!" I said.

He shrugged and picked up his spoon. "It is what it is."

"Was anyone else at home?" David asked.

"Nah, just me." He dug into his bowl of soup. "My

wife died a year ago, and my only son . . . he killed himself last month."

After a few beats of silence, he looked up. Glancing from my shocked face to David's, he smiled faintly. "It is what it is." Then he went back to eating.

You never know where you'll run across a philosopher. In this case, we were in the cafeteria of a physical-rehab facility.

A week earlier, as David reclined his wheelchair all the way back, its controller had gone blank. In spite of a fully charged battery, the chair had no power. I poked buttons, checked cables—everything I could think of. Finally, I brought his manual wheelchair up from the basement. From lying almost flat to getting out of the power chair sideways made for a challenging transfer, but we did it.

Then David got busy on the phone.

Calls to various departments of the VA added up to a total strikeout. Recordings, voice mails, no callbacks. We've had excellent experiences with the VA, but this was the exception. After that, we called local wheelchair businesses, but none had power chairs to rent. "We used to," one manager told us. "But they came back so torn up, we were losing money."

That made sense. But such a basic need! At least we had the manual chair, but I had to push him everywhere. This meant loss of independence for both of us.

Finally, my Nextdoor phone app found a neighbor willing to sell a power chair his aunt had used. We bought it. Smaller and lighter, the chair handled differently than what David was used to, but it worked. We celebrated with a chiminea fire on our patio that evening and stayed out late. Night was taking over by the time I scooped the dying coals into the fire bucket and carried it into our garage.

"Help!"

The word came from outside the garage, muffled but unmistakable. I ran back out to the patio. The temporary chair stood upright—and empty. No David in sight. I looked wildly around. "Where are you?"

"Here."

I tracked his voice. "What are you doing under the elderberry bush?"

In the growing darkness, he'd missed the path and run one wheel up onto a brick at the edge of the patio wall. The chair tossed him onto the flagstones and righted itself. He rolled under the elderberry.

Call 911, ambulance to the ER, hospital

admittance—we'd been that route before. After about a week, David shifted to the rehab facility with the philosopher whose bruised face matched David's shoulder and torso.

As I drove home alone that evening, leaving David in his small, impersonal room, my mind went back to our lunchroom conversation. *It is what it is.* The phrase fit the way I felt about our current situation. Sad, tired, wishing I'd never bought that chair, but mostly just resigned to slogging through this setback.

Sometimes, we need lots of words. We need to pour out pain, grief, fear, anger, discouragement—or a tangled mix of them all—to someone who will listen. But other times, we don't need that. Instead, it seems right to accept what's happened and settle in to do what must be done. No need to weep or fret. This season of affliction is simply part of life, and after a while, we'll leave it behind. That's the way life works for everyone.

In this world you will have trouble.

It is what it is.

28

IT'S MORE
THAN IT IS

In this world you will have trouble. But take heart!
I have overcome the world.

JOHN 16:33, NIV

CERTAIN MOMENTS TOUCH US MORE powerfully than
the events themselves can explain. I'd never known
what to call those times. Then I read Colossians 1:20
in *The Message.*

> Not only that, but all the broken and dislocated
> pieces of the universe—people and things,
> animals and atoms—get properly fixed and fit
> together in vibrant harmonies.

Vibrant harmonies. I love that.
Our neighbor across the street, a caregiver for his

wife, hung a bird feeder beside their front door. Birds and squirrels came and went, leaving seeds and shells scattered across the porch floor. Every evening, Eric swept the mess away. I walked by one day and made some silly comment about his housekeeping skills.

"Oh, Janet likes birds." He gestured toward the glass storm door. "She sits in the living room all day and watches them. That's why I put the feeder here."

Nice, right? That's what I thought. But the next time Eric came out with his broom and began sweeping, the patience and constancy of this service to his wife pierced me with its beauty. As Janet's illness worsened, she had less and less to enjoy. This was Eric's gift to her.

A piercing beauty. A vibrant harmony.

David and I moved to Colorado Springs in June. Every morning for two months, we took our coffee to the front porch, where we sat and talked until it was time to go to work. Then came the bicycle accident. Much of this blurs for me, but I know I spent that first night and the next day at the hospital. Late that afternoon, David's parents and both of his sisters arrived. I came home to shower, then went back to the hospital for the night.

Early the following morning, I drove home. I brewed

a pot of coffee and carried my cup out to the front porch. This would be my first morning here without David, and I felt strange and shaky.

His sister Susan was awake. She poured herself some coffee and came to join me.

That made all the difference. I don't remember our conversation, but I do remember feeling connected, relaxed, *right*. Over the next few days, we would all rely on Susan's experience as a nurse to interpret what we saw and heard at the hospital. Her knowledge and competence were invaluable. But those moments on the porch had nothing to do with that. This was her being herself and us being together.

A restful peace. A vibrant harmony.

Two years after David went back to work, a new teammate moved into the next cubicle. Bret helped David stand and walk, emptied his leg bag, got his lunch from the fridge, refilled his water jug—whatever needed to be done. They joked about Bret being David's armor-bearer.

One day, David seemed unusually quiet when I picked him up from work. On the drive home, he told me Bret had asked our boss to change his job description to include helping David. They pulled up his paperwork and made the addition. "So, it's official," Bret had said, smiling but serious.

"When he told me that, I felt honored." David had tears in his eyes. "And I felt protected. It's so hard, not being able to do things for yourself and always having to ask."

A deep comfort. A vibrant harmony.

Caregiving makes a perfect breeding ground for such moments. Vibrant harmonies are relational, and so is caregiving. We human beings will never be perfect until heaven. But sometimes we get a glimpse of what that looks like.

29

KEEP A LOW CEILING
AND A HIGH FLOOR

You're allowed to have a seat, and you're allowed to have a voice,
but . . . you are absolutely forbidden to drive.

ELIZABETH GILBERT, Big Magic

THE DAY AFTER DAVID'S ACCIDENT, our daughter and
her friend signed us up for a CaringBridge site. This
allowed me to sort through all that was happening and
write about it online. People could find out how we
were doing and express their love and concern. They
also posted advice, some of which I appreciated more
than others.

One of the best suggestions, "Keep a low ceiling and
a high floor," arrived from a friend while David was
still in the critical care unit (CCU). What great timing
that was.

During those two weeks in the CCU, his condition

fluctuated like a roller coaster with no one at the controls. "You'll never move again," a doctor told him. A few days later, David raised and lowered each foot. Then he couldn't. Then he could. He wiggled the fingers of his right hand. An X-ray showed pneumonia in one lung—"It's bad. Full of gunk." The meds cleared it up. After a week and a half of trying, he finally moved one finger of his left hand. Then he got pneumonia again.

Celebrate! Grieve. Rejoice! Worry. David's family and friends were all on that roller coaster with him. I was trying to listen to God, but I could barely hear through the wind shrieking in my ears.

Then came our friend's suggestion. Her explanation was brief but clear, and the phrase "a low ceiling and a high floor" created an image that stayed in my mind.

Instead of the spike-and-plunge chaos of a speeding roller coaster, imagine you're walking down a long, quiet hallway that stretches into the future. All those contrary emotions still go with you, but now they travel in a gentle up-and-down curve. No neck-jerking highs and lows.

As this new word picture slowed me down and quieted the mental commotion, I could think more clearly. I could wait. Emotions had less power to take over and haul me along. I could lean on God and look toward the next step.

David noticed the change. When he moved the other fingers of his left hand, I was happy but didn't burble on about him "getting everything back." When Craig Hospital had no open bed for him, I expressed disappointment but treated this as the temporary setback it proved to be. I told David about low ceiling and high floor, and he tried it too. He liked it. We used this concept in the CCU, at Craig Hospital, and after we came home. It covers all areas of life, including children, finances, and plumbing problems.

This may sound like a contradiction of what I said earlier about facing our fears, asking ourselves, *What's the absolute worst that could happen?* But the craziness of a speeding roller coaster isn't the place for that. A quiet hallway is. We're no longer terrified, devastated, or furious. We *are* still scared, hurt, or angry.

But now we can also think.

30

CATCHING A
DOWNDRAFT

We recover from broken limbs, not amputations.

JERRY SITTSER, A GRACE DISGUISED

"BLIND CLIMBER SCALES MOUNT EVEREST!"

"Quadriplegic Woman Sails Solo Across the English Channel!"

"Blind Quadriplegic Flies Biplane Around the World!"

No, that last headline isn't real. But the other two are. And Erik Weihenmayer and Hilary Lister make up only a tiny percentage of the handicapped people tackling crazy challenges like those. If you Google "amazing things disabled people have done," you can spend hours reading the results.

Feel like an underachiever? This should make you feel better.

David and I don't even do overnight road trips.

We used to travel a lot, much of which involved camping. We loved it, but now the risks and hassles outweigh the fun. "Handicapped friendly" motel rooms that aren't. The mountains of supplies I have to pack in the van, then carry into and out of those unfriendly rooms. And most important of all, David's vulnerability to compression fractures. Long car rides are hard on him.

Compared to Erik and Hilary, that sounds pathetic. But it's our choice. We don't travel.

Because of this, David rarely uses his vacation days, and one of our teammates got onto him about that. "You need time off," she said. "At least a day or two now and then."

So David blocked off one Monday a month on his work calendar. We both got excited about the idea.

The first vacation Monday came in October, sunny and warm with a crisp autumn breeze. A long, perfect, leisurely day stretched out in front of us. We could do anything we wanted.

It was miserable.

For the first time in years, the contrast between pre- and post-accident life hit us in a deep, wrenching, emotional way. Before, we would have turned this into a long weekend, packing our tent on Friday evening and driving to the mountains. We would have hiked, cooked out, sat around the campfire. I hadn't cried about David's physical situation in a long, long time, but that day I did. I almost wished we didn't have the memories from before. They made this life look small and sad.

I have lost much.

You have lost much. Right?

If you're like me, you mostly do okay with that. But sometimes, it's as if you're flying along, minding your own business, and suddenly hit a downdraft. Crash and burn. The source of your downdraft might be obvious—like our not-so-fun vacation day—or you might see no reason at all. Just a random downdraft.

I came across a quote that expresses this well. "Occasionally, weep deeply over the life that you hoped would be. Grieve the losses. Feel the pain. Then wash your face, trust God, and embrace the life that he's given you."[1]

We live in a culture that likes to tell us how we should live, think, and even feel. Unless someone asks a direct question about travel, I don't volunteer the information that we never do. If they do ask, I tell them. Then they often say something like "I know a guy who's a quadriplegic, and he and his wife go skiing in Switzerland."

Well, good for him. Good for his wife. That's not David. That's not me.

There are benefits to staying home. My neighbor knows I'm always available to feed his cats if he goes out of town. I can take care of our garden myself instead of finding someone to water it. David and I sit on the patio to enjoy the flowers and talk and drink coffee and watch the birds. Sometimes we walk-and-roll around the neighborhood. Friends come over. Family members visit from out of town. We listen to music or read.

Occasionally, we grieve the losses. Because we *have* lost much.

Then we embrace the life we have.

31

FROM METAPHOR TO REALITY

The quickest way for anyone to reach the sun and the light of day
is not to run west, chasing after the setting sun, but to head east,
plunging into the darkness until one comes to the sunrise.

JERRY SITTSER (FROM HIS SISTER, DIANE),
A Grace Disguised

"THEN WASH YOUR FACE."

That's the bridge in the center of the quote I like so much: "Occasionally, weep deeply over the life that you hoped would be. Grieve the losses. Feel the pain. Then wash your face, trust God, and embrace the life that he's given you." Those four words stand as the transition between looking back at what we've lost and moving toward what we have in its place.

It's a good metaphor. But how do we turn that into reality? What does "washing your face" look like?

A Grace Disguised, a rich, deep, honest book, came out of Jerry Sittser's experience of losing his mother, wife, and daughter to a drunk driver. I treasured and learned from the whole book, but one section surprised me.

"Sorrow," Sittser writes, "is noble and gracious. It enlarges the soul until the soul is capable of mourning and rejoicing simultaneously. . . . However painful, sorrow is good for the soul."[1]

Is it? Sorrow can rip and twist the soul, leaving it in bitter shreds. It can numb the soul, so a person is never fully alive again. It can turn people against God, so they never trust him again. I've seen all of that happen. But for sorrow to be good for the soul, maybe "washing your face" is an essential step.

Sittser writes about a night when his young son expressed anguish and rage, wanting to make the drunk driver suffer as he'd made their family suffer. Sittser held him, and they sat in silence. Then his son said, "You know, Dad, I bet someone hurt him, too, like maybe his parents. That's why he did something to hurt us. And then I bet someone else hurt his parents. It just keeps going on and on. When will it ever stop?"[2]

Listen to those words! You can hear sorrow enlarging that child's soul. He hadn't reached the place of rejoicing, but he was edging onto that road. He had begun to look beyond himself, beyond the now.

In that story, I saw four parts of "washing your face":
Be with someone you trust.

Talk honestly. Express your feelings.

Allow yourself times of silence, making room for truth to shift within you.

If there's a place for forgiveness, forgive.

During that worst-vacation-day-ever, when grief for what we'd lost knocked David and me for an unexpected loop, we talked it out. We didn't try to solve or fix anything. We just expressed. Some parts we went into more deeply or from a different angle than ever before, and I had a sense of *something* happening in me.

My soul, enlarging? A bridge, leading me to trust God more than before?

For Sittser, "washing his face" doesn't mean denying his grief. He doesn't leave sorrow behind. He takes it with him and allows it to coexist with the joy he finds in life. I don't know how to do that, but I don't think he did either. Not at first.

We learn along the way.

32

WORTH THE LIMP?

Jacob named the place Peniel (God's Face) because, he said,
"I saw God face-to-face and lived to tell the story!"
The sun came up as he left Peniel, limping because of his hip.

GENESIS 32:30-31

"I'M TIRED, FEEL LIKE A HOPELESS FAILURE, have lost the energy necessary to be cheerful and strong as I deal with David's needs. Instead of resting in God, I often have that squeezed, anxious feeling in my chest that I remember from the first week after David's accident.

"He's worried about me. I'd be worried about me if I had enough energy."

This little burst of sunshine comes from my journal of 2014, the year I would rather not remember. Everyone has a year like that.

Ours began with David strapped into a clamshell brace, recovering from two compression fractures. Then a publisher got excited about my first novel, *Safe*—which got me excited, too—but her committee totally and squashingly rejected it. About that time, David's mild nerve pain ballooned and intensified, and his ability to move diminished. An MRI tracked the cause to thickening scar tissue in his neck. As we looked into surgery for that, another compression fracture buckled his leg and threw him down the three steps to our back door. While he was in the hospital, a close relative attempted suicide.

Enough, right? We're less than halfway through the year, but you don't want to hear the rest any more than I want to tell it.

Instead, fast-forward to the long-awaited joys of September, when four of us old high school friends had a reunion in beautiful Cape May. Back home, David's delightful, capable sister Jean had arrived to take over his caregiving for the week. After two years of caring for terminally ill homeless people, she should have no trouble dealing with David. I could relax and enjoy. Talk, eat, wander along the beach, poke around the little shopping area, crank open the striped awning of our cottage's front porch and lounge in its shade. Talk more. Eat more. Relax. Enjoy.

But I *couldn't* relax, couldn't fully enjoy this idyllic vacation. In normal life, I rarely cried, but it happened several times that week. On the last day, tired and tense, I had a major meltdown over a minor disagreement.

I flew home in deep discouragement. Though David had urged me to go on this trip and worked out details to make sure I could, I knew my absence was tough on him. And Jean's demanding job made it unlikely we could do this kind of swap again. As I'd kept telling myself, this was probably my only chance for a vacation like this. And now I'd wasted it.

Why? What went wrong?

Looking through my 2014 journal, I see a pattern in how I named that year's events. *Hard. Scary. Exhausting.* Then the word "too" started showing up, as in *too hard, too scary, too exhausting.*

In other words, too much to handle. Overwhelming. Impossible. My own words tipped me over the edge, and the safety net of a vacation in Cape May couldn't bear up under the force of my fall. Nothing could have.

This is one of those lessons I've had to learn more than once. Years earlier, I'd been struck by what Jacob named the site of his wrestling match in Genesis 32. He could easily have called it "Permanent Limp," since he'd arrived there whole but left with a disability. Instead, he named it "God's Face," saying, "I saw God face-to-face and lived to tell the story!" And Jacob himself got a new name there. From being Jacob, or "Deceiver," he became Israel, or "God-Wrestler."

Worth the limp? He thought so.

Instead of calling 2014 "The Year I'd Rather Not Remember," what if I name it "God Strengthened and Deepened Me"? That's exactly what took place through that hard, scary, exhausting year, though it wasn't obvious at the time. It felt more like the opposite. But looking back, I can trace the changes.

Worth the pain? Oh, yes.

If you've been thinking about your year like that, I hope you'll see what was happening for you then. And let's both hope we've learned our lesson once and for all.

33

TELL IT LIKE IT IS

The storms of love are not calmed by magic, but by facing
them in faith and going through them.

PETER SCHMIDT, *How Did Love Become a Reality Show?*

"JILL!"

My response came instantly. Hunched-up shoulders, scrunched-up eyes, clenched-up stomach. As my body parts slowly unknotted themselves, I took a deep breath and called, "Coming!"

This had been my strongest reaction so far. Strong enough to prod me into finally acknowledging its cause.

First, I dealt with what David needed from me. Then I told him, "I'm starting to hate the sound of my name."

"You are?" he said. "Why?"

"Because it always means either you want something, or there's a problem. It's never a happy thing."

David and I do marriage mentoring as part of our job, and I know enough not to use dynamite words like *always* and *never*. But this time, they were accurate, although David didn't think so. Not until he caught himself doing exactly what I'd said over the next few days.

"You were right," he said.

How I love those three words!

After that, I started hearing statements like "Jill! I love you," or "Jill! You look great today." Not a perfect balance, of course. His accident was still recent, and he had many needs and problems. But David kept working to change the trend, and his efforts paid off. Just having him take me seriously helped as much as the words themselves.

I used to think of assertiveness as a form of aggression—being pushy and demanding, even bullying. But the online marriage assessment David and I use gives couples a thumbs-up for scoring high on assertiveness. "It's really just being honest with each other about what you want," David tells them. "Having freedom to do that indicates a healthy relationship."

True for marriage, and true for caregiving. Since his accident, David and I have had plenty of those honest moments.

I realize this could be a hard topic for you. The way David responded might be poles away from what you experience. Maybe your person isn't mentally or physically capable. But you might have other family members in the picture who could use a good dose of assertiveness.

The other day, I came across *New Dawn New Day New Life*, a blog by Kristen, who cares for her quadriplegic husband. In one post, "I'm a Caregiver and a Wife and a Mother—Here's What I Want," she wrote about finally getting honest with her husband and their daughter.

"I'm always asking, 'What do you need? What do you want?'" she told them. "No one ever asks *me* that question."[1]

It's a good blog, candid and well written, and I love the way the story ends. You should read it. I appreciate how she expressed her anger but didn't let it take over. In the long run, what she said could have a deep impact for good. Not just for her but for the people she loves.

That's what we really want, isn't it?

My honesty opened David's eyes to a habit he disliked in himself as much as I did. What if I hadn't spoken up? Unhealthy dynamics build up momentum, and they rarely stop on their own. Or if I'd waited too much longer, addressing the issue might have looked less like assertiveness and more like a nuclear blast. Loud and destructive.

David has done the same for some of my blind spots. Although I never like that, I need it. I'd rather hear the words "You were right" coming out of *his* mouth, but saying them myself is good for the soul.

Tips on confronting:

- Wait until you're not tired or angry.

- If you have several topics, choose one and stick with it.

- Instead of criticizing, say, "This is what I want."

- Make your explanation brief and digestible.

34

STEPPING BACK

The unexamined life is not worth living.

SOCRATES

THIS MIGHT BE A GOOD PLACE to step back and consider how being a caregiver has changed you. Every book needs a quote by a Greek philosopher to give it a touch of class, and I chose "The unexamined life is not worth living," by Socrates. Severe, maybe, but that shows he felt strongly about this.

Some of my changes lean toward beauty. With others, affliction stands out. My list begins with:

- In being stretched emotionally and physically, I've become stronger. *Beauty.*

- I have less time and freedom to build friendships.
  Affliction.
- Music goes in deeper than it used to. *Beauty.*
- Having experienced my power to shame David,
  I hate it and am determined to never use it again.
  Affliction that has turned into beauty.

That's a good one to stop and think about. I've talked about the need for caregivers to give shame no chance to latch on and drag along behind us. But if we caregivers are vulnerable to shame, how much more is that true of our person? As David said of his teammate's willing help, "I felt protected. It's so hard, not being able to do things for yourself and always having to ask."

We can protect our dignity in ways our person can't. We see them at their weakest, often when we're tired or stressed. It's easy to slide into shaming.

Step back. Step away. Turn around. Move toward being safe for your person. We can't erase what we've done, but we can change.

After writing those words, I went downstairs, took a deep breath, and asked my husband, "Do I ever make you feel ashamed?"

He thought for a moment. "No."

Whew. Beauty.

I didn't want to ask, but I needed to. "Is there anything else I do that you wish I wouldn't?"

More thought. "Yes."

Affliction.

That led to a lengthy conversation about the way I'd been overcorrecting David. "By the time we go to bed," he said, "some days, I feel I didn't do *anything* right. I know that's an exaggeration, but . . ."

But he was right. Lately, I'd had an uneasy awareness of speaking up too often and with impatience. "Why didn't you . . .?" "I've asked you not to. . ." Assertiveness is good, but balance is essential. And impatience has strong ties to shaming.

Don't let me go that way, God.

Step back. Keep changing.

35

THE LAST ELEPHANT

End of construction—Thank you for your patience.
RUTH BELL GRAHAM'S EPITAPH

EVERY CAREGIVER I'VE MET HAS REGRETS. I do, and I'm sure to collect more.

So does every ex-caregiver whose person has died. Almost without exception, they talk of piercing regrets about the last days or hours of their person's life. They say, "I should have . . ." or "I shouldn't have . . ." But it's almost certain that if they *had* done what they now regret not doing, they would now regret having done that. And if they hadn't done it, they would now regret not doing it.

If that doesn't make sense to you, don't worry. Regret itself is a riddle. How can something be sharp, dull, heavy, and empty all at the same time? Why would we forget where we just parked the car, but be dogged by every detail of a long-ago failure? Does regret never die of old age?

When a pair of earrings kept bringing up a grievous regret from years ago, I told a friend. She scolded me for dwelling on the memory and said I should hand it off to God. I told another friend. She said it wasn't a big thing, and I shouldn't let it bother me.

Then I told David. He listened and asked a few questions.

Finally, I said, "I'm going to pack these earrings away. That won't undo the past, but I don't need the constant reminder."

"Good idea," he said.

Here's the crazy part: Since I talked with David, the regret has lost its oomph. I still keep those earrings in my jewelry box and see them every day. I even wear them occasionally. Good memories from around that time have floated up to take over from the one that tormented me.

I didn't expect that, but I'll accept it.

Regrets are inevitable. We're still under construction, incomplete and imperfect. Caregivers have plenty of opportunities to make mistakes, and some of mine have had sizable consequences. We can't know everything, and we can't do everything exactly right. Some choices are a toss-up. Sometimes nothing we do will make a difference. But afterward, we blame ourselves anyway.

We could think of regret as the fourth elephant, but it's more like a mosquito with an oversized shadow, whining and bumping against the window screen. We learn from failures. We see God redeem them. They give us compassion and understanding to pass on to others. And they don't define us.

Those regrets are not who you are. *This* is who you are:

Beauty and affliction.

God's hands.

Quiet hero.

A strand in the safety net that couldn't be complete without you.

YOU'RE STRONGER THAN YOU THINK.

ACKNOWLEDGMENTS

This was the hardest page of all to write. I don't want to leave anyone out, but I owe so much to so many, there's no way to fit you all in.

First, of course, many thanks to my beloved husband, David. Not only is he the whole reason for this book, but he kept me going whenever I whined that I didn't like writing nonfiction because I couldn't just make everything up.

I want to thank Don Pape, who first got the book rolling at NavPress, and David Zimmerman, who took the baton with the same quality of heartwarming encouragement and professionalism. Elizabeth Schroll's copyediting made revisions easy. And I'm thankful to others on the NavPress and Tyndale team whose roles have been less obvious to me but equally important.

My writers' critique group went through every word of every chapter with me, sometimes more than once, raising questions, encouraging, and prodding. So, thank you to Jani Dick, James Hart, Heidi Likens, Carol Reinsma, Mark Sellers, and Faye Spieker. (I put too many commas in this paragraph, right?)

Penrose Hospital in Colorado Springs, Craig Hospital in Denver, and the VA Hospital in Aurora have saved David's life, improved its quality, and given me training and tools to be his caregiver.

Other caregivers have spent much time answering my questions. Thanks especially to Brenda and Melinda, the two women whose stories you'll find on the next pages.

Finally, thanks to family and friends. David and I need you all.

OTHER PEOPLE'S STORIES

If you're caring for someone with dementia, our caregiving experiences are vastly different. Even so, we also have much in common, and I hope some of these stories and the principles underlying them connected in a helpful way. Here are two stories from other caregivers that might have meaning for you.

Brenda

The human heart has hidden treasures,
In secret kept, in silence sealed.

CHARLOTTE BRONTE, "EVENING SOLACE"

I know Brenda through a friend. We've never met in person, but our email connection went deeper than usual in a short time. She said writing out her story and thinking about my questions helped her make a significant move forward. After I sent her the quote I like so much ("Occasionally, weep deeply . . ."), she's the one who came up with the question of what it means to "wash your face."

❧

Some people say I'm a tough nut to crack. They're only half right.

My father left when I was young. I watched my mom struggle, and that was it for me. I would *make* life happen—I would take care of myself. I joined the Air Force at eighteen and stayed with the military for thirty-seven years. Believe me, it was hard being a woman in that life. Many times I cried, bled from my heart, and was on my knees to God.

I thought *that* was tough. Now I know God was preparing me for a much tougher journey.

Four years before retirement, I met Mike. Kind, sweet, and respectful, he melted my heart. We were both in our early fifties, and neither had ever married. That changed in June 2011, on a special day that touched the hearts of many who came to watch us exchange vows.

During our first month of marriage, Mike got lost coming home from work. One simple change in the subdivision where we lived threw him off completely. Once I got him home, I realized something was going on. I texted his brother to ask if he'd seen any deterioration in Mike when he came for the wedding.

He said yes.

I knew Mike had suffered a severe brain injury in a car accident two years before we met. I'd never seen any warning signs while we were dating. Now I did . . . and I had just taken a vow to be there for him, no matter what, in front of God, family, and friends.

Things got worse. I was terrified. I was angry with God. No longer a tough nut, I had become a broken bride dealing with the reality of losing her love. When we finally got Mike's diagnosis of early-onset Alzheimer's, he became my total mission in life. I enrolled him in adult day services, where healthy challenges—field trips, service animals, music therapy—let him stay home longer than he could have otherwise. I called the local Presbyterian church to ask for a Stephen Minister, a lay person trained to walk alongside someone in crisis. What a tremendous help for our journey.

My toughest day in military service was nothing compared to the day I had to place Mike in a care home an hour away. He'd gotten worse, and I'd worn out. By then, we had been married five years. I prayed for wisdom and guidance. I lost weight, didn't sleep, and lived with pain like a sword in my heart. I wept before God and held tight to him.

I visited Mike four or five times a week. It would have been seven, but they told me to pace myself because the worst was yet to come. One day, he could no longer feed himself. He lost the use of his legs, became incontinent, couldn't speak. I hated watching what this disease was doing to him. Unlike a lot of people with Alzheimer's, Mike understood what was going on. I told him our marriage *wasn't* a mistake. This tough nut had become more tender, more gentle, more understanding, more kind, and more loving because of him and this disease.

Those last days, I would walk into his room and say, "Kisses for heaven! Who wants kisses for heaven?" Then I would give him tons of kisses. I told him, "You can give one to Jesus and save the rest till I get there."

The best days were when he remembered how to kiss me back. I thanked him for giving me kisses for earth to keep in my heart.

When the time came, I cried with sadness and joy. At the age of fifty-nine, the love of my heart was finally home free.

I'm thankful I kept my vows. Mike needed someone like me to be a strong advocate in his disability, and I'd learned how to do that in the military. But God knew I needed Mike more than he needed me.

Mike was God's special nutcracker to change me.

Melinda and Harold

The beauty of a thistle.

CAROL REINSMA

Melinda is the sister of one of our teammates. She was open and honest and gave our phone call as much time as we needed. I hope to meet her someday.

❧

"The last year of Mom's life," Melinda said, "I was sitting in her room one day. She was in bed. She looked at me with tears in her eyes and said, 'I wish you could just sit in here with me and just be with me all the time.'

"That was really hard. I held her hand and said, 'I do, too, Mom.'"

As we talked on the phone, Melinda's awareness of emotions amazed me. They were scattered throughout her story, rich, clear, and useful. She could pinpoint how she felt at different seasons of caregiving. She also recognized the feelings that still pulled at her.

"When I think back," she said, "I feel guilty about all the emotional ways I didn't support Mom. She needed love and physical touch. A gentle, caring touch different from just dealing with the necessities. Every day, I held her hands, gave her kisses, told her how much I loved her. I could tell it meant a great deal to her. I'm so thankful I did that."

When Melinda and her husband first brought her to live with them, her mom had recently lost a leg to diabetes. Between that, dementia, and congestive heart failure, no one expected her to live more than three years.

"Harold and I talked about that before we said yes. I know it sounds calloused, but I was working full-time. Harold had retired, so we knew much of the caregiving would fall to him. Mom could go to adult daycare three days a week, but Harold would be on duty the other two. He was willing. We decided we could do this for three years."

Melinda is familiar with caregiver fatigue. Her mother woke her several times each night, calling her name, wanting to be taken to the bathroom. Going to her full-time job provided a break of sorts, but it also meant she came home tired and went straight into caregiving.

"In the evenings, Mom wanted to come into the living room with us, but sometimes I just wanted time alone with Harold. I felt so selfish. But her dementia meant there could be no real conversation. Every day, she asked me the same questions over and over. Sometimes I just didn't want to deal with that.

"I felt so much during those years. Sad, overwhelmed, exhausted, loving. And I constantly felt torn between my mom and my husband. He's older than I am, and I kept thinking of all the time we were missing together. How many more years would I have with him?"

Her mom's death, after seven and a half years, brought a sense of sorrow and release. "It wasn't that

I wanted her to die. I loved her. I *wanted* to be her caregiver. But she had a lot of pain, especially the last two years. And I wanted normal life. Time with my husband.

"Harold was my strength—I couldn't have done it without him. And my sister Robin came almost every other weekend. It was good to have the break from caregiving, but it was also fun just to have her here, something positive to look forward to. Robin and I could laugh over silly things no one else would find funny.

"This has changed me. It increased my compassion for people who are helpless like my mom. She didn't ask for this to happen to her. I have more empathy for those in my position too. I have a caregiver friend who calls when she needs to talk about what's going on with her. And now, another friend whose husband got early-onset Alzheimer's calls me. She tells me, 'I had no idea what you were going through with your mother.'

"The years with my mom were hard," Melinda said. "And I'm thankful for them."

Questions for Reflection and Discussion

The following are questions to facilitate personal reflection and group discussion. The chapter that the question most naturally relates to is included with the question.

How do you feel about your role as a caregiver so far? (chapter 1)

What are your stories of beauty? Of affliction? (chapter 3)

How do you feel about the idea of being part of a safety net? (chapter 3)

How did your caregiving story begin? (chapter 4)

How has carrying this burden changed you? (chapter 5)

Does your burden ever feel overwhelming? What do you do about it? (chapter 5)

Who are the people you look to as an example in your journey as a caregiver? Why them? (chapter 6)

Have there been areas of false hope you've had to give up? What were they? (chapter 7)

Have you had seasons of denial? What did that look like? (chapter 7)

Who are the quiet heroes in your caregiving story? (chapter 8)

Are you free to take care of yourself? Why or why not? (chapter 10)

How do you discern the balance between taking care of yourself and taking care of your person? (chapter 10)

What do you find especially difficult to be thankful for? (chapter 11)

How has fatigue affected you as a caregiver? How often are you operating out of fatigue? (chapter 12)

Do you see yourself getting stronger? How? (chapter 12)

Body, mind, will: In which of these do you most experience fatigue? (chapter 13)

Do you see what you're doing as important? Why or why not? (chapter 14)

How have you seen small tasks make a difference for your person? (chapter 14)

How does the possibility of your person dying affect you? How, if at all, would you like to change that? (chapter 16)

How do you make tweaks to your routine? (chapter 19)

How do you feel about the idea that it's reasonable to sometimes wish your person would die? (chapter 21)

How do you give your person feedback on their efforts? (chapter 23)

Are there areas that are particularly hard to be patient about? (chapter 23)

Do you find yourself feeling angry with your person? What is usually at the root of your anger? (chapter 24)

Do you have any areas of creative outlet? What are they? (chapter 25)

What's the balance between "It is what it is" and "I need to talk to someone"? (chapter 27)

What aspects of your situation do you find difficult to accept? (chapter 27)

What moments of vibrant harmony would you like to tell people about? (chapter 28)

How do you respond to the idea of low ceiling, high floor? (chapter 29)

Have you seen sorrow enlarge your soul? (chapter 31)

To what extent are you able to express what you want? How do you handle it when your person expresses what they want? (chapter 33)

How has being a caregiver changed you? Name the beauty and the affliction. (chapter 34)

NOTES

3: CONNECTING
1. "Caregiving in the U.S. 2020," National Alliance for Caregiving, accessed September 23, 2021, https://www.caregiving.org/caregiving -in-the-us-2020/.

9: TOTALLY UNQUALIFIED
1. *American Heritage Dictionary*, 2nd ed. (1976), s.v. "hero."

11: THE RIGHT KIND OF ADDICTION
1. For example, see Julia Guerra, "16 Benefits of Gratitude, According to Science and Mental Health Experts," Mind Body Green, updated September 10, 2019, https://www.mindbodygreen.com/0-6823 /10-Benefits-of-Gratitude.html; and Steve Scott, "31 Benefits of Gratitude: The Ultimate Science-Backed Guide," Happier Human, August 1, 2020, https://www.happierhuman.com/benefits-of -gratitude/.

13: DIVIDE AND CONQUER
1. John Ortberg, *Soul Keeping: Caring for the Most Important Part of You* (Grand Rapids, MI: Zondervan, 2014), chap. 11.

14: WELL-KEPT

1. *The Joy in Living: A Guide to Daily Living with Mother Teresa*, comp. Jaya Chaliha and Edward Le Joly (New Delhi, India: Penguin Books, 1997), 137.

17: CLIMB IN THE CAR

1. Bekah DiFelice, *Almost There: Searching for Home in a Life on the Move* (Colorado Springs: NavPress, 2018), 148.
2. "What Is a Stephen Minister?" Stephen Ministries, accessed September 2, 2021, https://www.stephenministries.org/stephen ministry/default.cfm/1596.

21: THE THIRD ELEPHANT

1. Nell E. Noonan, *The Struggles of Caregiving: 28 Days of Prayer* (Nashville: Upper Room Books, 2011), 40.

22: IT CAN HAPPEN

1. "Lifesaving Naloxone," CDC, accessed September 23, 2021, https://www.cdc.gov/stopoverdose/naloxone/?s_cid=DOC_Naloxone_PaidSearch_028.
2. "Odds of Dying," National Safety Council, accessed September 23, 2021, https://injuryfacts.nsc.org/all-injuries/preventable-death -overview/odds-of-dying/.
3. "Benzodiazepines and Opioids," National Institute on Drug Abuse, accessed September 23, 2021, https://www.drugabuse.gov/drug -topics/opioids/benzodiazepines-opioids.

30: CATCHING A DOWNDRAFT

1. John Piper, "Embrace the Life God Has Given You," Desiring God, March 10, 2017, https://www.desiringgod.org/embrace-the-life -god-has-given-you.

31: FROM METAPHOR TO REALITY

1. Jerry Sittser, *A Grace Disguised: How the Soul Grows through Loss* (Grand Rapids, MI: Zondervan, 1995, 2004), 74.
2. Sittser, *A Grace Disguised*, 75.

33: TELL IT LIKE IT IS

1. Kristen, "I'm a Caregiver and a Wife and a Mother—Here's What I Want," *New Dawn New Day New Life* (blog), January 31, 2020, newdawnforus.blogspot.com/2020/.

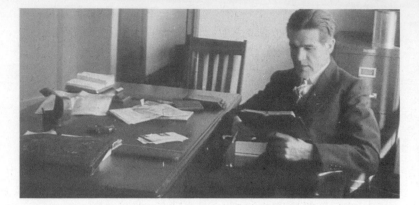

THE NAVIGATORS® STORY

———————— ⟨⟩ ————————

T HANK YOU for picking up this NavPress book! We hope it has been a blessing to you.

NavPress is a ministry of The Navigators. The Navigators began in the 1930s, when a young California lumberyard worker named Dawson Trotman was impacted by basic discipleship principles and felt called to teach those principles to others. He saw this mission as an echo of 2 Timothy 2:2: "And the things you have heard me say in the presence of many witnesses entrust to reliable people who will also be qualified to teach others" (NIV).

In 1933, Trotman and his friends began discipling members of the US Navy. By the end of World War II, thousands of men on ships and bases around the world were learning the principles of spiritual multiplication by the intentional, person-to-person teaching of God's Word.

After World War II, The Navigators expanded its relational ministry to include college campuses; local churches; the Glen Eyrie Conference Center and Eagle Lake Camps in Colorado Springs, Colorado; and neighborhood and citywide initiatives across the country and around the world.

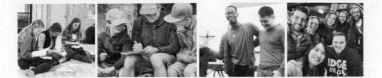

Today, with more than 2,600 US staff members—and local ministries in more than 100 countries—The Navigators continues the transformational process of making disciples who make more disciples, advancing the Kingdom of God in a world that desperately needs the hope and salvation of Jesus Christ and the encouragement to grow deeper in relationship with Him.

NAVPRESS was created in 1975 to advance the calling of The Navigators by bringing biblically rooted and culturally relevant products to people who want to know and love Christ more deeply. In January 2014, NavPress entered an alliance with Tyndale House Publishers to strengthen and better position our rich content for the future. Through *The Message* Bible and other resources, NavPress seeks to bring positive spiritual movement to people's lives.

If you're interested in learning more or becoming involved with The Navigators, go to navigators.org. For more discipleship content from The Navigators and NavPress authors, visit thediscuplemaker.org. May God bless you in your walk with Him!

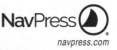

navpress.com

CP1308